Alternative Medicine
and Spinal Cord Injury

Alternative Medicine and Spinal Cord Injury

Beyond the Banks of the Mainstream

Laurance Johnston, Ph.D.

New York

Demos Medical Publishing, LLC, 386 Park Avenue South,
New York, New York 10016

Visit our website at www.demosmedpub.com

With permission from the publisher, much of the information in
this book was adapted from an ongoing series of articles published
in *PN/Paraplegia News* magazine.

Library of Congress Cataloging-in-Publication Data

Johnston, Laurance.
    Alternative medicine and spinal cord injury / Laurance Johnston.
        p. cm.
    Includes bibliographical references and index.
    ISBN 1-932603-50-6 (alk. paper)
    1. Spinal cord—Wounds and injuries—Alternative treatment.
    2. Spinal cord—Wounds and injuries—Patients—Rehabilitation.
    3. Alternative medicine.   I. Title.
    RD594.3.J646 2005
    617.4'82044—dc22   2005006521

Printed in Canada.

The purpose of this book is to provide information to readers
so that they can make more informed decisions about their
own healthcare. It should not be construed as medical advice
and readers should always consult with their doctors.

Dedication

This book is dedicated to the Paralyzed Veterans of America (PVA), whose assistance and association over the years have been greatly appreciated. Although I have worked for some of the nation's foremost public-health agencies, none have had more heart and soul than PVA.

Edmund Burke, the 18th-century English philosopher, stated: "*Society is a contract.... It is a partnership in all science, a partnership in all art, a partnership in every virtue and in all perfection. As the ends of such a partnership cannot be obtained in many generations, it becomes a partnership not only between those who are living, but between those who are living, those who are dead, and those who are to be born.*"

By building on the contributions of those who have gone before with a commitment to future generations, PVA has always demonstrated a commitment to this social contract.

Contents

Foreword

Alternative therapies have traditionally faced great bias from the biomedical community. However, they should not automatically be discounted because they don't fit into traditional medical thinking.

Certainly, researchers need to open-mindedly carry out well-designed clinical trials to generate scientific proof for new treatments for spinal cord injury (SCI), but alternative therapies may help some people who have SCI.

In an effort to inform subscribers about these nonmedical treatments, *PN* magazine created the column Healing Options as a vehicle for disseminating Dr. Johnston's articles. Carefully researching each topic, Dr. Johnston has, over the years, described a wide spectrum of alternative modalities. His articles have generated kudos as well as condemnations. On the one hand, they have concerned some members of the medical community, who adamantly panned the concepts. On the other hand, many readers responded with heartfelt thank-yous.

Alternative therapies may not help all people all the time or even some people all the time, but they may aid some people some of the time. The most important thing is that the information has been available. This book has consolidated many of his *PN* articles, as well as other material, into an informative, easily readable resource for individuals with SCI, health professionals, and others interested in SCI healing options.

Cliff Crase
Editor, *PN* Magazine

Acknowledgments

There are many individuals I wish to thank for support over the years and whose contributions at some level contributed to the book's evolution.

Foremost, I acknowledge many PVA colleagues, including (1) Cliff Crase and Ann Santos of *PN* magazine for creating the Healing Options series, which laid the foundation for the book; (2) my former boss and friend John Bollinger; (3) Thomas Stripling and the Education Foundation Board of Directors for funding my efforts to expand the healing spectrum; and (4) Mountain-States Chapter colleagues who published my first foray on this subject in their newsletter.

I am also deeply thankful for many scientific mentors, including Dr. Francis Neuhaus, Northwestern University (IL) and Olaf Runquist, Hamline University (MN); and the numerous teachers of alternative and mind–body–spirit healing wisdom who shared paradigm-expanding insights with me, including Almine Barton, Countess of Shannon.

I am grateful for my many mentors with physical disabilities, including Dr. David Gray, who shared with me the heart and soul behind disability, which sometimes is lost in detached policy-making.

I am also appreciative of many policy-making colleagues, including my former supervisor Dr. Duane Alexander, Director, National Institute of Child Health and Human Development, who provided invaluable opportunities to learn about the creation of disability programs at a national level.

In addition, I am thankful for the friendship of Audur Gudjonsdottir, Iceland's 2002 Woman of the Year, who shares with me a vision of what is possible after SCI if we open-mindedly integrate divergent pieces of the puzzle that exist throughout the world.

Finally, I am indebted to my parents, Scott and Laura Johnston, as well as Jean Lindahl, for support at many levels.

Preface

This book provides information on alternative and complementary therapies that can expand the healing spectrum for individuals with spinal cord injury (SCI). It discusses healing perspectives and paradigms that have not been a part of traditional modern medicine but that, nevertheless, comprised a key component of healing armamentaria throughout much of mankind's history. The various subjects are frequently discussed from a holistic, mind–body–spirit view, in contrast to conventional medicine's reductionistic orientation that views us as a sum of our body parts whether molecules, cells, organs, or a spinal cord, which can be repaired in isolation.

In spite of the focus on alternative medicine, this book does not try to negate modern medicine's many valuable contributions, which cumulatively have greatly extended the life expectancy of individuals with SCI. Most healing traditions have something valuable to offer yet, at the same time, have limitations in scope. Modern medicine emphasizes important pharmacologic and surgical approaches; however, other healing traditions stress often equally valid, but different therapies that medicine has traditionally ignored (for example, until recently, nutrition). It is as if medicine looks at the world through red-tinted lenses, and other disciplines green, blue, or yellow lenses. Unless we work together more in unity than opposition, each discipline's vision will remain inherently limited. However, if we open-mindedly accommodate divergent views of what is possible, we create an expanded healing spectrum that will benefit all, including those with SCI.

Although it is often assumed that modern medicine represents safe, proven therapies and that alternative medicine does not, nothing could be further from the truth. In fact, only a small fraction of routinely used conventional therapies (including those representing SCI medicine) are scientifically proven, and, furthermore, through adverse side effects, medical mistakes, and antibiotic-resistant infections, conventional medicine has a downside that can inordinately affect those with SCI. This book provides some wellness-enhancing alternatives that will reduce exposure to this downside while at the same time increasing medicine's power when truly needed.

The book is divided into sections that represent diverse healing approaches. Following an introduction that reviews why alternative medicine has become so popular in recent years, chapter 2 discusses Traditional Chinese Medicine's acupuncture and qigong and India's ancient Ayurvedic healing tradition. Chapter 3 focuses on laser therapy's potential to restore some function and treat SCI-associated hand problems. Chapter 4 reviews various natural and vibrational healing therapies, including homeopathy, herbal medicine, aromatherapy, flower essences, and Edgar Cayce's SCI approaches. Chapter 5 covers various bodywork approaches, such as chiropractic and craniosacral therapy. Chapter 6 discusses thought-provoking dolphin-assisted healing, and chapter 7 reviews electromagnetic healing. Chapters 8 and 9 move into mind–body–spirit healing modalities, including indigenous Native-American medicine and the role of prayer, spirituality, and consciousness. Chapter 10 reviews naturalistic approaches to enhance urinary tract and prostate health, fight diabetes, and build strength. The last chapter discusses inert-gas therapy, a healing modality that incorporates many paradigm-expanding concepts.

With the support of the Paralyzed Veterans of America, this book is the product of many years of effort researching various alternative healing modalities. Considerable time was spent reviewing each topic, including interviewing many leading experts. Although much of the material was initially published in some form in *PN/Paraplegia News*, a widely circulated magazine in the disability community, this volume for the first time integrates this extensive material into a readily assessable and readable resource. While it will benefit virtually anyone who wishes to learn more about alternative medicine, it especially targets individuals with SCI, their families, friends, caregivers, and health-care providers.

Laurance Johnston, Ph.D.
Boulder, CO

1

Introduction

The 19th-century German philosopher Arthur Schopenhauer stated: "Every man takes the limits of his own vision for the limits of the world." The purpose of this book is to provide information on various alternative, complementary, or energy-based therapies that provide a different "vision for the limits of the world," and by so doing, expand the healing spectrum for spinal cord injury (SCI). For the sake of simplicity, these therapies hereafter will be collectively called alternative medicine.

Given the book's emphasis, it is important to note that professionally I am a product of the mainstream biomedical establishment. For example, my doctorate is in biochemistry and molecular biology; and I was an FDA regulatory official, a National Institutes of Health (NIH) division director, and a director of Paralyzed Veterans of America's (PVA) Spinal Cord Research and Education Foundations. As I began to review and study divergent healing concepts as a result of PVA funding, my strongly held beliefs on the supremacy of modern biomedicine started to crumble. As it did, I was able to see a world of opportunity beyond the banks of the mainstream.

The therapies discussed in this book not only have the potential to help a variety of SCI-aggravated problems, but they also have the ability to restore appreciable, quality-of-life enhancing function. A number of chapters will summarize alternative healing disciplines and their relevance to SCI, and other chapters will review various alternative clinics or programs targeting SCI. The book's overall purpose is not to advocate alternative over conventional medicine, but to expand the healing spectrum available to individuals with SCI, in turn allowing them to make more informed decisions about their own health care.

Before we start to discuss various alternative approaches to healing, we need to address some of the reasons that such approaches should be considered and dispel some myths about their use, especially relative to conventional allopathic medicine.

REASONS FOR ALTERNATIVE MEDICINE'S POPULARITY

Although people with SCI have benefited greatly from modern medicine, like millions of other Americans they are concerned about the adverse consequences of technology-based medicine and desire health care with a more holistic perspective. Modern medicine focuses on fixing the symptoms, often ignoring the underlying mind–body–spirit causes. Under the pretext of scientific objectivity and reductionism, medicine detaches itself from the patient's uniqueness and operates by isolating and fixing the dysfunctional item in the absence of the big picture.

In contrast, many alternative healing traditions have more of a holistic view that focuses on disease causes and not merely on symptoms. Because most illnesses have mind–body–spirit contributions, effective health care should consider all three. In spite of many breakthroughs, conventional medicine often has limited perspectives, especially when it comes to chronic health issues. For example, although nutrition is probably the most important factor to long-term health, most medical schools do not require a course in nutrition.

Dr. Wayne Jonas, former director of the NIH Center for Complementary and Alternative Medicine, summarized some of the reasons for the surge in popularity of alternative medicine (1), including

> a rise in prevalence of chronic disease, an increase in public access to worldwide health information, reduced tolerance for paternalism, an increased sense of entitlement to a quality of life, declining faith that scientific breakthroughs will have relevance for the personal treatment of disease, and an increased interest in spiritualism. (p. 1616)

He also notes that there is growing concern about the adverse effects and escalating costs of conventional care.

DEFINITION

Depending on one's viewpoint, alternative medicine definitions can vary greatly. For example, in the United States acupuncture is an alternative therapy, but in China it is traditional medicine. Face-tiously, consumers define alternative medicine as therapies they paid for out of their own pockets but did not feel comfortable discussing with their physicians. In contrast, physicians define it as quackery because it was not a part of their medical school curriculum.

Dr. Daniel Eskinazi proposed that alternative medicine be defined "as a broad set of health-care practices (i.e., already available to the public) that are not readily integrated into the dominant health-care model because they pose challenges to diverse societal beliefs and practices (cultural, economic, scientific, medical, and educational)" (2).

TRENDS

Because of consumer demand for health care options, there has been incredible growth in alternative medicine. Dr. David Eisenberg et al. reported that 40% of Americans used alternative therapies in 1997 (3). Between 1990 and 1997, visits to alternative practitioners jumped 47%. Over that same period, Americans visited alternative providers 629 million times compared to 386 million visits to primary care physicians. Ninety percent of alternative medicine users are self-referred (4); that is, they are educating themselves and not relying on traditional medical authorities.

Although the medical establishment frequently criticizes alternative healing, many rank-and-file physicians desire additional training in alternative therapies. For example, one survey indicated that 49% of primary care physicians want homeopathy training (5). Although curriculum content is uncertain, the majority of medical schools now offer some training in alternative medicine (6); and as health care consumers, 39% of family physicians use herbal remedies (7).

INDIVIDUALS WITH DISABILITIES

This grassroots movement seems especially true for people with disabilities, even in spite of their traditional reliance on conventional health care. According to analyses of the 1999 National Health Interview Study (personal communication, Dr. Gerry Hendershot, November 2, 2001; 8), they are using alternative medicine even more than able-bodied individuals are. For example, adults with a disability are $1\frac{1}{2}$ to $2\frac{1}{2}$ times more likely to use prayer or spiritual healing for health care than are adults without a disability.

FIRST, DO NO HARM

It is often assumed that conventional medicine has been proven safe and alternative medicine has not been. This assumption is false. Although modern medicine's many contributions have greatly benefited people with SCI, it also has a downside that inordinately affects them. Examples include the following:

- Annually, 106,000 people die from adverse drug reactions in hospitals, making it the nation's fourth to sixth leading cause of death (9). Painkillers alone, which people with SCI often rely on, hospitalize more than 76,000 people each year because of gastrointestinal complications (10). (In comparison, herbal remedies kill 50 to 100 people a year.)

- Almost 2 million people who enter hospitals in this country get infections they did not have when they went there. Of these, 80,000 die (11).

- According to the National Academy of Sciences, medical mistakes kill 44,000 to 98,000 people annually (12).

- Finally, studies suggest that hospital care in general rates as the third major killer in the country, following heart disease and cancer (13).

These statistics are especially relevant to people with SCI, who often are prone to overmedication, life-threatening infections, and more hospitalization. Clearly, such statistics warrant a serious consideration of alternative therapies, such as those summarized in this book.

DOUBLE-BLIND OR DOUBLE STANDARD

Although it is true that many alternative therapies have not been well tested, the prevailing assumption that conventional medicine represents scientifically well-tested procedures is inaccurate. For example, the Congressional Office of Technology Assessment (as well as others) concluded that only 10% to 20% of conventional medicine techniques have been scientifically proven (14). The double standard was underscored by a prestigious National Institutes of Health (NIH) Consensus Conference when discussing acupuncture (15). The conference concluded, "While it is often thought that there is substantial research evidence to support conventional medical practices, this is frequently not the case . . . the data in support of acupuncture are as strong as those for many accepted Western medical therapies" (p. 13).

ENERGY MEDICINE

One key feature that is often inherent in ancient or Eastern healing traditions and characterizes numerous alternative healing traditions is the concept of energy. Many scientists are beginning to explain energy concepts through an emerging mind–body discipline called psychoneuroimmunology. This is a long word for a simple idea: basically, your emotions, attitudes, and consciousness affect your physical health by releasing beneficial neurological agents, hormones, and immune-enhancing substances. An example of this is meditation, which produces profoundly beneficial physical effects. For example, those who meditate visit doctors half as much as those who do not; have lower rates of cancer, heart disease, and substance abuse; and age more slowly.

Although disciplines like psychoneuroimmunology are beginning to bridge the gap, historically there has been a huge philosophical difference between conventional medicine and energy-based healing traditions. Medicine's mechanistic perspective assumes the body's biochemistry is paramount, whereas the energy model believes that the biochemistry is subordinate to the body's energy. As discussed by Dr. Roberta Trieschmann (16, 17), conventional medicine assumes that physical health produces happiness and therefore considers emotional reactions, meaning of life, and belief systems to be irrelevant to medicine. In the energy model, happiness leads to physical health, and thus our beliefs, the meaning we attach to daily events, and our emotional reaction to these events are crucial to health and well-being.

MEDICINE AS A PREVAILING PHILOSOPHY

Many alternative healing traditions emphasize the role of spirituality or consciousness. In contrast, modern medicine is based on a mechanistic view of the body. Within this view, the body represents a summation of individual parts (molecules, cells, organs, etc.), and as a result must be healed by fixing the parts. Under such a model, spirituality or consciousness has no relevance to health.

Dr. Daniel Eskinazi states that under conventional medicine's materialism philosophy "physical matter is the only fundamental reality, and that all beings and processes and phenomena are manifestations or results of matter" (p. 1621). He argues:

> As it has not been demonstrated that physical matter is the only reality, materialism, therefore is akin to a religion, i.e., a system of beliefs held to with ardor and faith. Western allopathic medicine, therefore . . . reflects the dominant philosophical belief system of the society in which it developed. (2, p. 1622)

FACTORS THAT KEEP ALTERNATIVE THERAPIES ON THE FRINGE

Economic

Our health care has been determined as much by economics, politics, and professional chauvinism as by objective science. These factors have created the most expensive health-care system in the world, which, in spite of its cost, is not that good compared to other countries. For example, in a 13-country comparison study, the United States ranked an average of 12th for 16 health indicators (13). Given that many individuals with SCI are at the lower rung of the nation's socioeconomic ladder, our costly, suboptimal health care disproportionately affects them, once again suggesting the consideration of cheaper, less risky, and perhaps more effective alternatives.

One key economic issue is the regulatory approval process. In view of the daunting economics needed to prove the safety and efficacy of any new treatment, few alternative therapies, regardless of merit, will survive the regulatory testing gauntlet. Basically, we have adopted a regulatory process that only works well for patentable therapeutics with large markets and deep-pocket financial sponsors (e.g., drug companies). Given that it often costs hundreds of millions of dollars to carry out the testing needed to bring a new medicine to market, the market size for many disabilities, including SCI, does not justify the expenditure and effort from a profit-generating view. Because many generic alternatives cannot be patented, economic incentives are lacking.

There are many examples of economic factors influencing the nation's health care that work against alternative therapies. For instance

- Physicians obtain most of their information on medicines from the profit-motivated pharmaceutical industry.

- The majority of medical consultants who advise public-health agencies have financial conflicts of interest with the drug industry that their decisions profoundly influence (18).

- There is a strong association between authors' published positions on drug safety and their financial relationship with drug companies (19).

- Drug advertising has increased a thousandfold in recent years (20).

- Drug companies spend an average of $13,000 a year on each U.S. physician to market their products (21).

Resistance by Organized Medicine

Many alternative treatments have a history of suppression by the allopathic medical establishment. For example, after acupuncture started to become popular in the 1970s, the American Medical Association (AMA) pressured the Food and Drug Administration (FDA) to ban acupuncture needles except for use in a research protocol. Control issues remain to this day. As another example, the NIH Consensus Conference mentioned earlier concluded that acupuncture should be used only after a patient has seen an MD, ignoring a training differential in which physicians can practice acupuncture therapy after 200 hours of training, whereas non-MDs must train 3 years in an accredited school of Oriental medicine.

In yet another example, the AMA—which was founded largely to fight homeopathy—did everything in its power to squelch the discipline. In spite of growing evidence, including double-blind clinical trials that support homeopathy's use, dogmatic opposition continues to this day as documented by a state medical board's revoking the license of a homeopathy-practicing physician.

In a final example among many, chiropractic historically has faced vociferous opposition from organized medicine. This opposition lasted until a 1987 federal antitrust ruling found the AMA guilty of a prolonged systematic attempt to undermine completely the chiropractic profession, often using highly dishonest methods.

Limited Scientific Perspectives

Traditionally, scientists downplay the importance of phenomena they cannot explain. However, if we learn anything from the lessons of history—such as the persecution of Galileo for proving that the Earth moves around the sun or the ridiculing of Ignaz Semmelweis for audaciously suggesting that physicians wash their hands—it is that today's state-of-the-art beliefs are tomorrow's anachronisms.

One of my most powerful personal examples of this phenomenon involves Sir Hans Krebs, who was awarded the 1953 Nobel Prize for elucidating core biochemical pathways and whom I met when I was a fledgling biochemist. He showed me a slide of a form letter he had received from the prestigious journal *Nature*, rejecting his seminal work for publication because of insufficient scientific merit. Today, as I write about therapies that frequently challenge the status quo, I often reflect on Krebs' rejection letter. If the father of modern biochemistry could be rejected by prestigious scientific authorities, I wonder what innovative, function-restoring therapies we are rejecting today. What amazes me is that condemnation is not limited to those who advocate the status quo. I have noted consistently that innovators who desperately want acceptance for their therapy are often the first to condemn someone else's innovation.

Many alternative therapies involve paradigm-expanding perspectives not well appreciated by bioscientists who feel that physiological phenomena must be explained through biochemical mechanisms they understand. For example, bioscientists dismiss homeopathy because it cannot be comprehended pursuant to traditional biochemical principles. Understanding homeopathy required physicists, who understood quantum physics, chaos and complexity theory, and so forth. Similarly, acupuncture's life-force *qi* energy was beyond the pale of Western scientific thought, yet it is now being explained through subtle electromagnetic-energy effects.

In addition, for many alternative therapies, the specific treatment is based on the patient's unique symptoms and not on the disorder by name. Nevertheless, in numerous studies scientists have ignored this underlying precept and have given the same intervention to all subjects in the treatment group instead of individualizing the treatment according to symptoms. When the results were ambiguous, they questioned the therapy instead of their methodology.

Research Funding

Although alternative therapies are often criticized for being scientifically untested, relatively little money has been provided for such testing. For example, the NIH National Center of Complementary and Alternative Medicine program for evaluating alternative modalities represents less than half of one percent of the NIH budget. Given alternative medicine's immense popularity, this is a huge budgetary discrepancy and makes one wonder how relevant NIH truly is to real-world health care. When Congress forced NIH to establish the center more than a decade ago, it was initially named the Division of Unconventional Medical Practices, which, considering the bureaucratic importance of acronyms ("DUMP"), suggested its relative NIH priority.

ARE WE GOOD WORLD CITIZENS?

Most of the world's population cannot afford high-technology Western medicine and often must rely on traditional or indigenous healing therapies. For example, Somalia's per capita health-care cost is $11 compared to $5,000 plus in the United States. If we are going to be good world citizens, concerned about other humans, we need to consider these economic health-care disparities when we develop policies for treating SCI. In view of such considerations, the World Health Organization has recommended that alternative, complementary, and indigenous medicine be integrated into national health-care policies and programs (22).

Conclusions

Most healing traditions have something valuable to offer, yet also have limitations. Conventional medicine emphasizes important pharmaceutical and surgical interventions that are especially useful in treating acute disease and in emergency care, whereas alternative medicine, by supporting wellness, is more suitable for dealing with the chronic ailments that increasingly plague modern society. It could be said that conventional medicine looks at the world through red-tinted lenses and alternative disciplines through green-, blue-, or other-colored lenses. Unless we work more in unity than opposition, each discipline's vision will remain inherently limited, which would be to the detriment of all. However, if we are open-minded and accommodate divergent views of what is possible, we create an expanded healing spectrum that will benefit all, including those with spinal cord injury.

REFERENCES

1. Jonas WB. Alternative medicine—learning from the past, examining the present, advancing to the future. *JAMA* 1998; 280: 1616–1618.
2. Eskinazi DP. Factors that shape alternative medicine. *JAMA* 1998; 280:1621–1623.
3. Eisenberg DM, Davis RB, Ettner SL, et al. Trends in alternative medicine use in the United States, 1990–1997. *JAMA* 1998; 280: 1569–1575.
4. Studdert DM, Eisenberg DM, Miller FH, et al. Medical malpractice implications of alternative medicine. *JAMA* 1998; 280: 1610–1617.
5. Ullman D. Homeopathy and managed care: managed or unmanageable. *J Altern Complement Med* 1999; 5(1): 65–73.
6. Med schools go alternative. *Natural Health*, January–February, 1999.
7. Pharmaton Natural Health Products (Ridgefield, Conn.) Survey of Physicians, 1998.
8. Hendershot GE. Mobility limitations and complementary and alternative medicine: are people with disabilities more likely to pray? *Am J Public Health* 2003; 93: 1079–1080.
9. Lazarou J, Pomeranz BH, Corey PN. Incidence of adverse drug reactions in hospitalized patients: a meta-analysis of prospective studies. *JAMA* 1998; 279: 1200–1205.
10. Lawrence R, Rosch PJ, Plowden J. *Magnetic Therapy: The Pain Cure Alternative*. Rocklin, Calif: Prima, 1998.
11. Fisher JA. *The Plague Makers*. New York: Simon & Schuster, 1994.
12. Kohn LT, Corrigan JM, Donaldson MS. *To Err Is Human: Building a Safer Health System*. Washington, DC: National Academy Press, 2000.

13. Starfield B. Is US health really the best in the world? *JAMA* 2000; 284: 483–485.

14. *Assessing the Efficacy and Safety of Medical Technologies*, Congressional Office of Technology Assessment, 1978.

15. National Institutes of Health Consensus Development Statement—Acupuncture, 1997. Available at: http://consensus.nih.gov.

16. Trieschmann RB. The energy model: a new approach to rehabilitation. *Rehabilitation Education* 1995; 9: 217–277.

17. Trieschmann RB. Energy medicine for long-term disabilities. *Disabil Rehabil* 1999; 21: 269–276.

18. Kassirer JP. Why should we swallow what these studies say? *Washington Post*, August 1, 2004: B03.

19. Stelfox HT, Chua G, O'Rourke K, et al. Conflict of interest in the debate over calcium-channel antagonists. *N Engl J Med* 1998; 338: 101–106.

20. Jobst KA. Complementary and alternative medicine: essential for the future of effective, affordable healthcare? *J Altern Complement Med* 1998; 4: 261–265.

21. Reported on National Public Radio, July 23, 2001.

22. *WHO Traditional Medicine Strategy 2002–2005*. Geneva, Switzerland: World Health Organization, 2002.

2

Eastern Healing

ACUPUNCTURE

Acupuncture has become a widely popular alternative therapy in recent decades. Studies suggest that it has considerable potential for treating problems associated with spinal cord injury (SCI), including, in some cases, restoring quality-of-life-enhancing function.

History

Although acupuncture is an ancient healing tradition, its transition to the West was slow. Sixteenth-century Jesuit missionaries first reported the therapy, and in the 1800s troops from Far East military invasions brought the procedure back to France. In 1825, Benjamin Franklin's great-grandson translated French work on acupuncture (1). However, after a flurry of interest, acupuncture receded from medical consciousness until President Richard Nixon went to China in the early 1970s. Soon after Nixon's visit, the American Medical Association (AMA) pressured the Food and Drug Administration (FDA) to ban acupuncture needles except for use in an investigational study.

Nevertheless, acupuncture's popularity grew. In spite of technically violating federal law, many states authorized its use, and schools and accrediting organizations were established. After 1 million Americans were using the procedure annually, the FDA finally reclassified acupuncture needles in 1996. Soon after, a prestigious National Institutes of Health (NIH) Consensus Conference endorsed specific acupuncture applications.

Treatment and Diagnosis

Acupuncture-related therapies stimulate specific skin points by the insertion of needles or the application of heat, pressure, or massage. Acupuncture is often combined with a variety of other Eastern therapies, such as herbal treatments, food and nutrition therapy, exercise, and meditation. The thin, usually disposable needles rarely draw blood, and any discomfort is mild.

The World Health Organization has listed more than 100 disorders that are amenable to acupuncture. Acupuncture works better at early stages of a disease or disorder before impaired body function progresses into organic or tissue damage. It is often a preventive measure to preserve good health. Adverse effects are rare.

Acupuncture emphasizes diagnosis. Because the Western name for a disorder has little diagnostic relevance, two patients with the identical disorder may receive different acupuncture treatments according to their specific energy imbalances. Diagnostic methods include patient observation, history taking, and touch. Examining the tongue and feeling the pulse are especially important. Evaluating the pulse is much more involved than in Western medicine. A yin pulse and a yang pulse are taken at three locations on each wrist, measured by deep- and light-touch pressure. Each of these 12 different pulses corresponds to a specific organ. When the pulse of each wrist is taken simultaneously, the relative differences indicate the body's energy balance with respect to specific organs.

Although both medical doctors and non-MDs practice acupuncture, nonphysician practitioners usually have had much more training. Specifically, physicians can perform acupuncture after 200 hours of training, whereas non-MDs must train for more than 3 years in an accredited school of acupuncture or Oriental medicine.

Dr. Claire Cassidy surveyed nearly 600 patients of Chinese medicine and found great patient satisfaction (2). For example, 87% of surveyed patients were very satisfied with their care, 91% with their practitioner, 70% were happy with the cost, and 91% report that their presenting problem had improved. In comparison, only 30% were satisfied with conventional biomedical care, 43% with their physician, and 26% with the price.

Eastern Origins

With origins in Taoist philosophy, acupuncture evolved from observing that disorders were associated with increased sensitivity in specific skin areas. These areas were consistently linked to a specific organ and followed a defined topographical pattern. These patterns, or meridians, serve as pathways for life-force energy called *qi* (pronounced *chee*). According to traditional theory, the body is endowed at birth with a fixed amount of qi that is then depleted through daily living and supplemented by energy from food or air. Energy imbalance is the cause of all illness; the absence of qi is death. Qi circulates throughout the body in a well-defined cycle, moving from meridian to meridian and from organ to organ.

Qi is characterized by the dynamic interaction of two antagonistic yet complementary energy forces called yin and yang, each of which includes a portion of the other (Figure 2-1). Yin, the feminine, is associated with cold, dark, passive, and that which is deep or hidden. In contrast, yang, the masculine, represents heat, light, active, and that which is on the surface. Yin and yang are constantly interacting and changing, and one never exists in isolation from the other.

According to tradition, all substances are formed from fire, water, earth, metal, and wood. Fire contains the most yang, and water the most yin. The elements are created or destroyed by specific cyclical interactions. For example, fire melts metal, metal cuts wood, wood covers earth, earth absorbs water, and water puts out fire.

To each element is assigned one yin and one yang organ. Under this model, a bad heart (a fire organ) will adversely affect the lungs (a metal organ), which will in turn affect the liver (wood). Each organ has a meridian associated with it that contains a series of

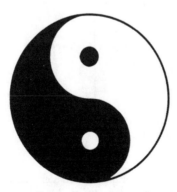

Figure 2-1 Qi is characterized by the dynamic interaction of two antagonistic, yet complimentary energy forces called yin and yang, each of which includes a portion of the other.

acupuncture points. Stimulating these points regulates energy flow in the meridians. Overall, it is a closed system in which the excess of energy in one area reduces the energy in another area.

Eastern medicine is interactive and holistic, that is, everything affects everything else. In contrast, Western medicine emphasizes component parts (e.g., kidney), often without seeing a relationship to the whole. The focus is on the symptoms, which according to Eastern medicine are merely the footprints left behind by energy imbalances.

According to traditional theory, traumatic SCI damages the Du or Governor meridian, which in turn affects yang energy of the entire body (Figure 2-2). The goal of treatment is to clear and activate meridian channels, reversing qi stagnation.

Scientific Basis

The NIH Consensus Development report on acupuncture stated the following:

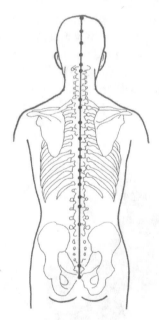

Figure 2-2 Du or Governor meridian, which is especially affected by spinal cord injury. Dots represent acupuncture points.

While it is often thought that there is substantial research evidence to support conventional medical practices, this is frequently not the case . . . the data in support of acupuncture are as strong as those for many accepted western medical therapies. (3, p. 13)

Although acupunctural theory is based on centuries of empirical, clinical observations, it was developed without modern physiological and anatomical insights. Because the idea of an intangible life-force qi energy flowing through anatomically undefined meridians seemed far-fetched to scientists and doctors trained in biochemistry, it was dismissed for many years. Effects were often attributed to heightened suggestibility, although such suggestibility could not explain how it worked in animals and infants. Scientists have now proposed numerous mediating physiological mechanisms to help explain acupuncture, including, for example, the following:

- Acupuncture stimulates neural pathways and neurotransmitter systems. For example, it stimulates muscle sensory nerves, which send messages to the spinal cord, midbrain, and pituitary, which in turn releases pain-reducing molecules called endorphins and cortisol-producing hormones (4). It has been shown in rabbits that the effects of acupuncture-induced analgesia can be transferred to other rabbits through the transfer of cerebrospinal fluid (5).

- Consistent with traditional representation of acupuncture points as energy vortexes, acupuncture points do indeed correspond to skin areas with unique anatomical and electrical properties (6). For example, an ohm meter placed over an acupuncture point will record greatly reduced electrical resistance compared to the surrounding skin.

- Through the release of specific molecules, acupuncture dilates blood vessels, thereby improving circulation.

Under traditional theory, all such physiological and molecular alterations are the function of changes in qi flow; that is, our biochemistry is subordinate to our energetic nature. Scientists have suggested that the body's qi energy can be related to very subtle bioelectromagnetic fields (7). Acupuncture perturbs these fields, and then these perturbations are magnified through more traditional physiological mechanisms. Although most living systems are sensitive to such subtle fields, the contribution of these fields to our biological understanding has been minimal because of difficulties measuring them and our emphasis on biochemical mechanisms.

ACUPUNCTURE AND SCI

People with SCI can benefit from acupuncture just as readily as able-bodied individuals. In addition, acupuncture provides a valuable treatment option for their unique health problems. Furthermore, evidence suggests that acupuncture has the potential to restore some function in both acute and chronic SCI. Virtually all chronic injuries have some intact but dormant neurons running through the injury site. Acupuncture may work by somehow turning on these dormant neurons. Animal studies suggest that only a small percentage of turned-on neurons are needed to have significant function.

The number of published studies focused on acupuncture's SCI benefits has grown considerably in recent years; several are summarized below:

- Gao et al. treated 261 individuals with SCI, of whom 79% had been injured at least 1 year (8). Ninety-five percent had some improvement, such as improved sensation, bowel and bladder function, spasticity, and walking. The authors speculate that acupuncture improves regeneration-promoting circulation around the spinal cord.

- Wang summarized the treatment of 82 cases of SCI with electro-acupuncture of bladder meridian points (lateral to the vertebrae) (9). Ninety-three percent accrued functional benefits, including improved lower-limb and bowel and bladder function.

- Cheng and colleagues showed that patients treated with electro-acupuncture achieved balanced voiding in fewer days than controls did (10). Patients starting acupuncture within 3 weeks of injury required fewer treatments compared to those treated later.

- Wong et al. treated acutely injured patients with electrical and auricular (ear) acupuncture starting in the emergency room and measured functional improvement 1-year postinjury with the commonly used ASIA (American Spinal Injury Association) assessment standards (11). Compared to controls, treated patients recovered more function.

- In eight patients with SCI, Honjo et al. demonstrated that acupuncture increases bladder capacity, decreasing urinary incontinence (12).

- Nayek and colleagues reported that 50% of acupuncture-treated patients with SCI had relief from chronic pain (13).

- Dyson-Hudson et al. found that acupuncture reduced chronic shoulder pain in wheelchair users with SCI (14).

- Rapson et al. treated with electroacupuncture 36 subjects who had below-level central neuropathic pain characterized by generalized burning. Twenty-four had reduced pain (15).

Anecdotal Stories

Artie's First Session

Artie, a combat-injured Vietnam veteran, was treated by acupuncturist Kelly for the first time. As is the case with many longtime wheelchairs users, Artie had chronic overuse problems with his shoulders and other areas. Although a wheelchair athlete who had recently ridden across Vietnam in a hand cycle, he was nevertheless initially apprehensive. Artie noted, "After years of being treated and analyzed by detached medical professionals, I was amazed how relaxed I quickly became. Kelly had a gentle, soothing style with an intuitive appreciation and understanding of the body. I didn't have to tell her; she quickly identified my sore-point areas. Furthermore, I was surprised that half the time, I didn't even know that the needles had been inserted. That night, my bad arm had no pain; I didn't even have to take my usual pills."

Jim's Story

"I am a 49-year-old Vietnam veteran. Due to depression resulting from posttraumatic stress combined with overmedication, I attempted suicide. I stuck a gun to my chest and shot myself. The bullet missed my heart and deflected off my sternum into my spine. My discharge summary reads T-12 SCI, permanent paralysis. After attending a wedding in Bolivia, I hooked up with a South Korean acupuncturist. I ended up having 30 days of inexpensive treatment and continued it back home. The speed at which I am rehabilitating is overpowering. Two weeks ago, I walked on a treadmill for almost 2 minutes (kafo on left leg and plastic afo on right leg). Presently, I can walk 45 feet with the kafo unlocked, assisted by a rolling walker. The improvement I have gained is a direct result of my acupuncture treatments."

Conclusions

Acupuncture has considerable potential to treat SCI-associated health problems, and in some cases to restore significant quality-of-life-enhancing function.

Additional Readings and Resources

Journal Articles

Naeser MA. Acupuncture in the treatment of paralysis due to central nervous system damage. *J Altern Complement Med* 1996; 2: 211–248.
Paola FA, Arnold M. Clinical review: acupuncture and spinal cord medicine. *J Spinal Cord Med* 2003; 26(1): 12–20.

Internet

Qi: The Journal of Traditional Eastern Health and Fitness: www.qi-journal.com
Acupuncture.com: www.acupuncture.com

SCALP ACUPUNCTURE

Scalp acupuncture is a specialized form of acupuncture that has helped many people with nervous-system disorders, including spinal cord injury (SCI).

Overview

Supplementing traditional body acupuncture, specific areas, such as the ear, foot, hand, and scalp, represent acupunctural microsystems for the entire body. Through treating a localized microsystem, health-enhancing energy flow, or qi, can be stimulated in virtually any body part.

Although the scalp acupuncture microsystem can treat most of the same disorders that traditional acupuncture does, it is especially effective in treating nervous-system disorders and pain. For example, studies have shown that scalp acupuncture has helped thousands of Chinese stroke patients, apparently through altering blood hormone levels that influence stroke-inducing platelet clumping. In addition, numerous people with multiple sclerosis, SCI, amyotrophic lateral sclerosis, and head injury have also benefited from scalp acupuncture. The therapy appears most effective when initiated soon after the traumatic injury or neurological crisis.

Spinal Cord Injury

One of the leading scalp acupuncturists is Professor Ming Qing Zhu of San Jose, California, who has authored many publications on the subject and has lectured internationally (16, 17). Over the course of his career, Zhu has treated many individuals with SCI. Although he emphasizes that scalp acupuncture is not a panacea, most of his SCI patients have accrued significant quality-of-life-enhancing health benefits, even though treatment was usually initiated long after acute injury, which is the most optimal therapeutic window. Even with chronic injuries, dramatic improvements can occur. For example, one patient with a T-11 gunshot injury came in for pain treatment and ended up regaining considerable walking ability.

Treatment

Very fine needles are painlessly inserted at a 15- to 30-degree angle into the thin layer of scalp tissue in treatment zones associated with specific body functions and regions (Figure 2-3). To stimulate qi flow, the needles are periodically manipulated. Because the needles are inserted in the scalp, the patient can receive treatment in any position, and the needles can be left in for extended, treatment-enhancing periods without interfering with daily activities. Typically, the needles remain inserted for at least the 2-hour clinic visit and often up to 72 hours.

In my case, I felt no pain when the needles were inserted and over time forgot they were there until I would absentmindedly run my hand through my hair. The needles didn't interfere with my

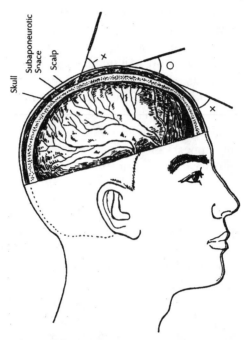

Figure 2-3 Very fine needles are painlessly inserted at a 15–30 degree angle into the thin layer of scalp tissue in treatment zones associated with specific body functions and regions. (From Zhu MQ. *Zhu's Scalp Acupuncture*. Hong Kong: 8 Dragons Publishing, 1992.)

sleep that night and were only pulled out the following morning because vanity required that I do something with my disheveled hair.

Physical Movement or *Daoyin*

An essential element of scalp acupuncture is *Daoyin*, physical and mental activities simultaneously carried out to direct the qi energy to affected body areas. Daoyin activities include chest and abdominal breathing, mental relaxation, massage, joint movements, pushing, pulling, rolling, standing, and others. Daoyin activities are customized to individual patient needs at the time of the treatment.

Basically, while the needles are being inserted, Zhu encourages patients to move the affected body parts or, at minimum, to visualize the movement accompanied with qigong-based breathing practices that help direct the qi flow to the intended area. He believes that such treatment-associated movement is critical in improving connections between the central and peripheral nervous system. Even with paralysis, Zhu encourages these movements, using assistive devices or the help of others as necessary.

Case Studies

At Zhu's clinic, I met Alessandro, an articulate, energetic 40-year-old quadriplegic with a charismatic smile and infectious enthusiasm (Figure 2-4). Before his injury, he led an active lifestyle that reflected his love of the outdoors. In 1997, Alessandro's life changed in an instant because of a renegade wave he chose to body surf. "A small 2-foot wave became an 8-foot face that took my 6-foot 2-inch, 215-pound body over the falls and dropped me headlong into the sand below...I immediately heard a crack...and knew under no uncertain terms that I was paralyzed." With his fifth cervical vertebrae now crushed, Alessandro notes, "What was once an active, adventurous outdoor lifestyle became an active, internal pursuit of recovery."

Alessandro believes that Zhu's care, treatment, and support was foremost in this pursuit, and feels Zhu is his "primary doctor." Alessandro says he fortunate to have been treated by Zhu initially only 12 days postinjury. "My initial treatment with Zhu in the hospital was not only

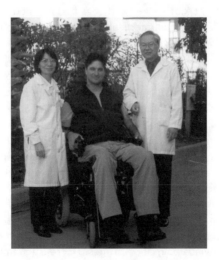

Figure 2-4 Professor Zhu and associate Moyee Siu with scalp-acupuncture patient Alessandro. (Photo taken by Laurance Johnston.)

incredibly and literally electrifying, but it really made me feel more at ease with my situation, physically, psychologically, and emotionally," he says. "Moreover, Zhu's therapy significantly aided in getting me off the pain pills I was taking as well as other drugs."

In spite of an original prognosis limiting his future activity to a "sip and puff" wheelchair, Alessandro has regained considerable function, which he attributes to Zhu's treatment, combined with his rigorous physical-therapy regimen. Alessandro has regained arm strength, some wrist control, and hand sensation, enabling him to use a phone handset and feed himself without a splint. Because he has also regained use of abdominal, lower back, and paraspinal muscles, he is almost at the point of doing unassisted weight shifts and lifting his torso upright in his standing frame. This additional torso strength has enabled him to sit for a long time while exercising on his mat table. For example, he can swing his arms back and forth in an exaggerated walking motion without assistance or falling over. Moreover, Alessandro says that Zhu's treatment has greatly enhanced his overall wellness, allowing him to direct his energy to functional recovery rather just attempting to stay well.

Tom, 21, sustained T-11 compression and T-12 burst fractures in June 2003. His MRI indicated a complete spinal-cord transection and severe spondylolisthesis. Classified as an ASIA-A injury (i.e., complete injury), Tom had neither motor or sensory function below the umbilicus nor bowel and bladder control. Seven months after initiating scalp acupuncture, herbal medicine, and a vigorous exercise regimen, Tom started walking with the assistance of walker and regained considerable bowel and bladder function. Defying all medical expectations, he progressed from ASIA-A to ASIA-C (partial motor and sensory recovery) in less than a year.

Nancy, 23, sustained a C5-7 incomplete injury from an April 2000 auto accident. Recovering in a Vancouver hospital, she solicited Zhu's assistance. A few weeks after injury, Zhu started treating her at bedside from morning to evening. Daily treatment typically began with both scalp and body acupuncture. The body needles were removed after 1 hour, but the scalp needles were left in for more than 24 hours. The bulk of the days consisted of almost nonstop exercises, from passive to active, the chest to the feet, the internal organs to external limbs, and lying to sitting positions. A little over a month after injury, she attempted to stand.

As Nancy recovered further, Zhu continued treatments, his main goals being to alleviate pain and soreness, increase stamina, correct posture and gait, and initiate new movements. Every week saw a small recovery breakthrough, which cumulatively resulted in Nancy's starting to walk with the aid of a walker by November.

Conclusions

Although the number of skilled practitioners is more limited, scalp acupuncture is probably more effective than traditional body acupuncture in treating SCI-associated problems and restoring some function.

Additional Readings and Resources

Books

Zhu MQ. *Zhu's Scalp Acupuncture*. Hong Kong: 8 Dragons Publishing, 1992.

Internet

Zhu's Scalp Acupuncture: www.scalpacupuncture.org

QIGONG

According to Traditional Chinese Medicine, a life-force energy called *qi* permeates all living things. Good health requires an ample and flowing supply of qi (pronounced *chee*). Depleted by demands of daily living, qi is naturally replenished through breathing, eating, and closeness to nature; it is deliberately enhanced by meditation, qigong, tai chi, and other principles of Traditional Chinese Medicine, such as acupuncture. When qi is consistently diminished, out of balance, or polluted, sickness ensues; its absence means death. Unfortunately, in people with a physical disability, qi can stagnate and become unbalanced, increasing the likelihood of illness. Therefore, it is especially important for them to stimulate qi flow.

Description

Influenced by a variety of Eastern spiritual philosophies over its 5,000-year history, qigong (pronounced *chee gung*) evolved to include medical, martial arts, spiritual, and, recently, business applications. China's government has been ambivalent toward qigong, sometimes encouraging it as a valuable homegrown healing tradition, and at other times viewing it as a counterrevolutionary vestige of the past. Because spiritual movements often force social change, the Chinese government cracked down on one qigong variation (Falun Gong) that stressed spirituality.

Qigong encompasses gentle movements, breathing, and meditative practices. According to author Kenneth Cohen (Figure 2-5), qigong "means working with the life energy, learning how to control the flow and distribution of qi to improve the health and harmony of mind and body" (18, p. 3) (Figure 2-6). It is a holistic, mind–body–spirit system of self-healing. Already one of the world's most popular healing exercises in terms of total practitioners, qigong is increasingly being embraced by health-conscious Westerners. Most qigong practices are relatively straightforward and easily mastered. However, because many different techniques exist, this chapter cannot provide in-depth specifics. Readers should look at the reference books listed at the end of this section.

With slight adjustments, most exercises are possible from standing, seated, or prone positions and, in the case of spinal cord injury (SCI), with or without arm movement. As such, qigong is an ideal activity for those with physical disabilities.

Key Elements

Posture and Relaxation

Qigong's relaxed, extended, open position enhances qi circulation. In this position, the joints are relaxed, the spine is straight and should feel long and extended, and the head feels as if it is suspended

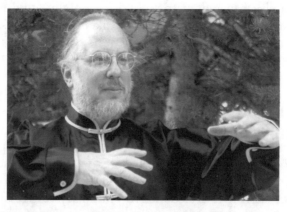

Figure 2-5 Qigong master and author Kenneth Cohen. (Photo provided by Kenneth Cohen.)

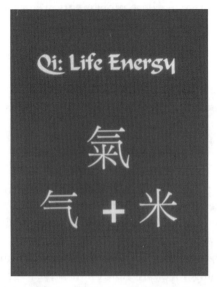

Figure 2-6 Combining two symbols creates the Chinese character for qi, the life-force energy. The left symbol represents steam; the right, rice. The combination signifies steam rising from cooking rice, indicating the importance of breath (i.e., steam) and food for replenishing qi. (Illustration provided by Kenneth Cohen.)

delicately over the spine. There is a sense of connection with the ground in which you feel as if your body weight is dropping or sinking through the feet.

Visualize any aspect that you cannot physically do. For example, "see" a straight spine or every part of your body sinking into the wheelchair and then into the ground. Scientists have shown that thinking about a movement can cause the same neurons to fire as actually doing it. Do not force movement, but rather use intent.

Breathing Practices

Qigong stresses deep, relaxed, abdominal breathing. Although paralysis often affects respiratory muscles, when you visualize this type of breathing, the benefits of qigong will still accrue and enhance your existing breathing capability.

Gentle Movements

Qigong emphasizes gentle, relaxed movements, closely integrated with breathing. Unlike more active exercise programs that stress strength and endurance, these movements are designed to promote energy flow, stimulating one's natural healing potential.

Self-Massage

Massage stimulates qi circulation, either locally for a specific area of pain or stiffness, or at a distant location—massage of the ears, hands and feet affects the entire body.

Meditation

Meditation, deep-relaxation, and visualization processes can have profoundly beneficial effects on mental state and in turn physical health. According to Cohen, individuals with a physical disability should emphasize meditation.

Cohen relates a poignant story about teaching a young man with SCI a qigong meditation. Cohen states: "After ten minutes the man began to cry, exclaiming that his legs were sweating for the first time since his car accident several years earlier. He could also feel some warmth in his legs" (personal communication, October 19, 1999). Cohen believes these meditations improve blood circulation and potentially repair damaged nerves.

Dr. Roberta Trieschmann, a preeminent SCI clinical psychologist and author, has incorporated qigong-related elements into her practice to improve the overall health and functioning of people with a physical disability. For example, by using these practices, an incomplete quadriplegic was able reduce his devastating central cord pain; and a woman who was legally blind because of multiple sclerosis was able to improve her sight enough to drive and read (19). "Both of these individuals were massively depressed by their circumstances and had lost all hope that life could be better for them," Dr. Treischmann says.

> Yet by understanding the role of energy in their life and changing the methods of managing their energy, they have been able to produce change in their function at the physical level even though a myriad of physicians could offer no hope for any improvement in their condition. (p. 269)

Qigong Science: A Blending of East and West

Qigong's healing claims do not lack scientific basis. For example, the Qigong Institute, in Menlo Park, California, has compiled a database of several thousand scientific studies documenting qigong's effectiveness in treating a wide variety of disorders (20).

Although historically dismissive of Eastern healing perspectives, many scientists are beginning to explain them through an emerging mind–body discipline called psychoneuroimmunology. This is a long word for a simple idea; basically, your emotions and psychological states affect your physical health. From a psychoneuroimmunology perspective, the qigong-induced mental states result in the release of beneficial neurological agents and hormones that strengthen one's immune system, which in turn fosters physical health. For example, qigong practice stimulates endorphin release, which is associated with moods of well-being or euphoria (e.g., the "runner's high"), and increases levels of DHEA, a steroid hormone associated with health and youthfulness.

Although the true nature of qi can only be speculated upon, scientists have shown that qigong-related practices can indeed generate a considerable amount of electromagnetic energy. Some believe that the qigong-associated energy induces hormonal shifts, by influencing the subtle electromagnetic fields that surround humans. In turn, these fields affect the brain's all-important pituitary and pineal glands, which secrete key hormones that regulate the entire body. These master glands have been shown to be sensitive to electromagnetic field fluctuations. Interestingly, a clustering of magnetic substances (called magnetite) has been found near these glands in an area called the Third Eye in Eastern healing and spiritual traditions. These traditions believe that this area is one of the body's most powerful energy centers—one that can be developed through qigong practice.

Consistent with ancient healing-tradition beliefs that Earth has a special, life-sustaining relationship with humans, Cohen feels that qigong exerts a healing effect by facilitating synchrony with the Earth's resonant, electromagnetic frequency. Cohen believes that such synchrony helps mitigate modern society's unhealthy electromagnetic pollution (e.g., computer screens, high-power lines, cellular phones, etc.).

Because of its gentle nature, anyone can practice qigong. And because disability inherently compromises qi flow, people with physical disabilities potentially can obtain more benefit from qigong than able-bodied individuals.

According to Cohen, "wisdom and wellness go together." He adds, "One cannot always expect a cure from qigong, but one can always expect some healing," defining a cure as a "measurable physiological change and healing as improved quality of life, happiness, and self-understanding" (personal communication, October 19, 1999). With this perspective, although physiological changes may be modest, improvements to quality of life may be profound.

SCI Meditations and Visualizations

Studies show that meditation can have beneficial effects on health. For example, meditators visit doctors half as often as those who don't meditate; have lower rates of cancer, heart disease, and substance abuse; and age more slowly. Many meditations involve some sort of visualization process. Qigong master Cohen suggests that individuals with SCI incorporate the following spinal cord visualizations into their meditations:

After assuming a comfortable position, close your eyes, take some deep breaths, and feel your muscles relaxing.

Meditation 1: Visualize a small ball of luminescent, white, healing light at your lower spine. Visualize this ball cutting through from this spot to your navel. From your navel, the ball rises up the front of your body and then goes over your head and down the back of your neck to about the C-7 cervical level. At this level, the ball of light cuts through to the front of your body. It then loops over the head again and goes down to next, lower vertebrate. Once again, the ball of light emerges through to the front of the body and loops over the head to the next vertebrate. The cycle is repeated until the tailbone is reached.

Meditation 2: Starting at the tailbone, visualize the ball of light traveling up your back on the outside surface of your spine. When it reaches the base of your skull, it enters the skull, circling up the inside surface of the back of your skull, around the top inside skull surface, and down the front inside surface behind your face. It then cuts over to your spine again, where it travels down the *front* of your spine to its bottom. At this point, visualize your spinal cord as a hollow tube in which the ball of light enters. The ball then travels up the *back* or *rear* of this spinal tube, and in turn proceeds around the inside of the skull as before. After entering the spinal cord again, the ball of light then travels down the *front* inside surface of the spinal tube. This represents one repetition. Do nine repetitions.

Conclusions

Whether explained through ancient Eastern philosophies or modern psychoneuroimmunology mechanisms, qigong enhances health and wellness, and expands our healing armamentarium.

Acknowledgment

Special thanks are given to Kenneth Cohen for assistance.

Additional Readings and Resources

Books

Cohen K, The *Way of Qigong: The Art and Science of Chinese Energy Healing*. New York: Ballantine Books, 1997.
Jahnke R, *The Healer Within: Using Traditional Chinese Techniques to Release Your Body's Own Medicine*. New York: HarperCollins Publishers, 1997.

Magazines

Qi: The Journal of Traditional Eastern Healing and Fitness (www.qi-journal.com)

Internet

Qigong Research and Practice Center: www.qigonghealing.com
The Qigong Institute: www.qigonginstitute.org

AYURVEDA

As the world's oldest known health-care system, Ayurvedic medicine is the granddaddy of healing traditions. Developed over centuries of use, it is a mind–body–spirit healing approach that attempts to keep people healthy and disease-free. Ayurveda's focus is the prevention of disease, including the sort of chronic health problems that frequently afflict individuals with physical disabilities, including spinal cord injury (SCI).

History

Ayurveda originated in ancient India more than 5,000 years ago. In spite, or perhaps because of these ancient roots, its influence in today's world may be greater than people think. For example, according to legend, Buddha, a great admirer of Ayurveda, sent teachers to different countries to integrate Ayurvedic insights into local healing traditions. These traditions in turn became the foundation for many of today's healing disciplines.

Ayurveda survived various threats over the millennia because it was deeply ingrained within Indian family customs and culture. These threats resulted in part from foreign conquests of India by Muslim nations and later the British, who imposed their medical standards (i.e., conventional medicine) on Indian society. After Indian independence in 1947, Ayurvedic medicine began to resurface and gain in popularity. The Maharishi Mahesh Yogi, transcendental-meditation program founder, facilitated its introduction into Western society. Ayurveda's visibility soared after the popular author Deepak Chopra began publishing best-sellers on the subject.

Theory

In Sanskrit, India's ancient language, *Ayurveda* means the science of life and longevity. It attempts to make sense out of life through living in harmony with nature. Because of its ancient origins, Ayurveda is explained with concepts and terminology developed without the benefit of modern anatomical and physiological insights.

People steeped in 20th-century medical thinking may view Ayurveda's tradition-based theories as archaic, with limited health-care relevance in today's world. Nevertheless, ancient wisdom often has much validity. Modern science increasingly is proving the effectiveness of many Ayurvedic therapies and approaches, and explaining how they work in modern scientific terms.

Ayurvedic Mind-Body Type

According to Ayurvedic theory, all individuals are made up of three basic energies, or *doshas*, called *vata*, *pitta*, and *kapha*. These are present in unique proportions defined at birth. Like a fingerprint, your characteristic mix, called *prakruti*, will distinguish you for life with respect to physical, mental, and emotional predispositions. It reflects your true, essential self. Although your prakruti, or energetic imprint, may be set for life, your day-to-day mix of vata, pitta, and kapha may vary greatly, depending how well you interact with your environment (e.g., stress, diet, exercise, and seasonal changes).

Your current mix is called *vikruti*. If your vikruti is identical to your prakruti (the Ayurvedic energetic imprint you are born with), your health should be excellent. Simply stated, if you can remain true to who you are from an Ayurvedic perspective, you will be healthy; if you cannot, you will invite disease.

The vata, pitta, and kapha doshas are associated with different individual characteristics:

Vata is the pranic life-force energy associated with physical and psychological movement, circulation, and the nervous system. People predominately influenced by the vata dosha tend to have thin, light, flexible bodies and are characteristically quick, change-able, unpredictable, enthusiastic, and talkative. They often possess quick minds and are creative. When out of balance, vata individu-als experience nervous-system disorders, energy or intestinal problems, insomnia, dry skin, and anxiety. The vata dosha is balanced by regular habits, quiet, attention to fluids, decreased sensitivity to stress, ample rest, warmth, steady nourishment, and oil message.

Pitta energy governs metabolism. Pitta individuals are often of medium height and build; and tend to be fiery, intense, possess a sharp and creative mind, a penetrating look in their eyes, a ruddy complexion, a competitive streak, and a hot temper. When out of balance, they experience fevers, inflammatory disorders, heartburn, ulcers, skin rashes, anger, and irritation. Moderation, coolness, leisure, exposure to natural beauty, and decreased stimu-lants balance the pitta dosha.

Kapha energy governs the body's structure and provides strength, vigor and stability. Kapha individuals usually have strong, large, healthy, well-developed bodies that tend to gain weight. They are even-tempered and calm, and have impressive endurance. When out of balance, Kapha individuals are predisposed to respi-ratory and congestion disorders, sinus problems, obesity, tumors, and lethargy. The kapha dosha is balanced by regular exercise, weight control, a variety of experiences, warmth, dryness, and reduced sweetness in food.

Balancing the Doshas

To maintain health, you must strive to adjust your vata, pitta, and kapha mix to match the Ayurvedic ideal you were born with. To do this balancing, you must know (1) your current mix of vata, pitta, and kapha (vikruti), reflecting your present state of health; and (2) your born-with Ayurvedic constitution (prakruti), reflecting what you wish to regain. In other words, you need to know where you stand now and what you are aiming for. These assessments can be obtained using questionnaires that are included in many Ayurvedic reference books.

Once you understand your doshic imbalance, you should take appropriate actions to help realign your mix of vata, pitta, and kapha in the desired direction. For example, although you may have been born with a kapha constitution, the stress of modern living and a fast-food diet has aggravated your vata dosha. As a result, you are now experiencing vata-associated disorders such as anxiety, insomnia, or intestinal problems. To remedy this imbalance, you would take steps to reduce vata aggravation and promote kapha expression.

In Ayurveda, these steps emphasize diet and nutrition, exercise, rest and relaxation, meditation, breathing exercises, medicinal herbs, and rejuvenation and detoxification programs. Modern science is increasingly recognizing the benefits of many of these lifestyle factors.

Holistic Sensory Therapy

In Western medicine, the five senses have little therapeutic role. For example, if you are given a drug, its taste or smell is not important. However, in Ayurvedic medicine, the senses play a key role because they are considered doorways to your internal physiology. As such, Ayurvedic therapies frequently attempt to evoke various sensory combinations. With this view, food and spices will trigger physiological responses not only through its nutrient value but also through taste and smell (Figure 2-7). Thus, with Ayurveda, the whole is greater than the sum of the parts.

For example, acquiring your vitamin C through freshly squeezed orange juice is more meaningful than a vitamin C supplement. In general, this approach reflects a major difference between Eastern holistic and Western reductionistic medical philosophies.

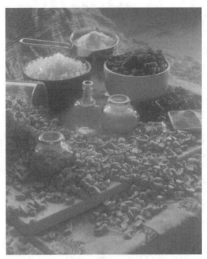

Figure 2-7   In Ayurveda, food and spices will trigger physiological responses not only through their nutrient value but also through taste and smell. (Photo provided by Maharishi Ayur-Ved Products, Colorado Springs, CO.)

Where Western medicine would attempt to isolate and then market a plant's physiologically active component, Ayurveda would use preparations of the whole plant. In addition to the active ingredient, Ayurveda believes that other synergistic components and sensory-provoking aspects of the plant are also important.

Diet

In Ayurveda, digestion is the foundation of good health. The doshas produce a metabolic fire, called *agni*, that transforms nourishment from food, feelings, and thoughts into a form your body can use. If your digestive fire isn't working properly because of doshic imbalance, you will produce toxins, called *ama*. Ama will clog both your body's physical (e.g., intestines, arteries, etc.) and nonphysical (e.g., energy) channels. To prevent ama accumulation, individuals should favor different types of foods depending upon whether they are more influenced by vata, pitta, or kapha doshas. According to Ayurvedic theory, the American diet aggravates the vata dosha, which has resulted in many of the health problems that characterize American society.

Ayurveda and SCI

People with spinal cord dysfunction often have an increased incidence of chronic health problems. These problems are aggravated by the considerable physiological and metabolic shifts that occur in the body after paralysis. From an Ayurvedic perspective, these shifts increase the divergence between the vikruti (the current mix of vata, pitta, and kapha) and the prakruti (the born-with vata-pitta-kapha ideal). For example, SCI promotes a vata imbalance. If this is not corrected, ama (toxins) will accumulate, clogging the body's channels and in turn causing disease. Hence, people with SCI need to be vigilant in their efforts to regain a good doshic balance, especially with respect to foods and behaviors.

Certain spices are recommended for clearing channels of ama after any sort of injury, including turmeric, black pepper, ginger, coriander, fennel, and licorice. According to animal studies, the Ayurvedic herb *Mimosa pudica* (the sensitive or touch-me-not plant) promotes neuronal health. Specifically, scientists have observed in rats with experimental injury of the sciatic nerve (which runs through the pelvis and upper leg) that regeneration was 30% to 40% higher in the animals treated with the *Mimosa pudica* extract (21).

I carried out a small pilot study testing the effects in paralyzed veterans of a multiherbal product containing *Mimosa pudica* (namely, "Re-Gen Nerve" from Maharishi Ayur-Ved Products (22). Twelve men and one woman with an average age of 52 were recruited, nine with SCI, two with multiple sclerosis, and one each with spinal meningitis and spinal cerebellar degeneration. Although no statistically significant functional improvements were noted as expected for a small pilot study of limited duration, subjects reported a variety of subtle effects (23).

Conclusions

Ayurvedic medicine represents an ancient health-care tradition that is becoming increasingly popular as an alternative medicine modality. Its emphasis on health maintenance through enhancing inherent healing ability has considerable relevance for many chronic health problems, including those that frequently afflict people with spinal cord injury.

Glossary

agni: the digestive fire that provides energy for the body to function

ama: toxic impurities that remain after improper digestion, which is the root cause of many diseases

dosha: the three forces (vata, pitta, kapha) responsible for determining an individual's constitution controlling the functions of mind and body

kapha: one of the three doshas; responsible for body structure

pitta: one of the three doshas; responsible for digestion and metabolism

prakruti: your inherent nature, as expressed by the proportion of the three doshas you were born with

vata: one of the three doshas; responsible for movement

vikruti: your current state; the ratio of the three doshas that fluctuates along with your health

Additional Readings and Resources

Books

Bruning N, Thomas H. *Ayurveda: The A–Z Guide to Healing Techniques from Ancient India*. New York: Dell, 1997.
Chopra D. *Perfect Health: The Complete Mind/Body Guide*. New York: Harmony Books, 1991.
Lad V. *The Complete Book of Ayurvedic Home Remedies*. New York: Three Rivers Press, 1998.

REFERENCES

1. Kaplan G. A brief history of acupuncture's journey to the West. *J Altern Complement Med* 1997; 3(Supplement 1): 5–10.
2. Cassidy CM. Chinese medicine users in the United States. *J Altern Complement Med* 1998; 4(1): 17–27.
3. National Institutes of Health Consensus Development Statement—Acupuncture, 1997. Available online at: http://consensus.nih.gov

4. Pomeranz B. Scientific research into acupuncture for the relief of pain. *J Altern Complement Med* 1996; 2(1): 53–60.

5. Han JS. Physiology of acupuncture; review of thirty years of research. *J Altern Complement Med* 1997; 3 (Supplement 1): 101–108.

6. Terral C, Rabischong P. A scientific basis for acupuncture. *J Altern Complement Med* 1997; 3(Supplement 1): 55–65.

7. Liboff AR. Bioelectromagnetic fields and acupuncture. *J Altern Complement Med* 1997; 3 (Supplement 1): 77–87.

8. Gao X, Gao C, Gao J, et al. Acupuncture treatment of complete traumatic paraplegia; Analysis of 261 Cases. *J Traditional Chinese Medicine* 1996; 16: 134–137.

9. Wang HJ. A survey of the treatment of traumatic paraplegia by traditional Chinese medicine, *J Chin Med* 1992; 12: 296–303.

10. Cheng PT, Wong MK, Chang PL. A therapeutic trial of acupuncture in neurogenic bladder of spinal cord injured patients—a preliminary report. *Spinal Cord* 1998; 36: 476–480.

11. Wong AM, Leong CP, Su TY, et al. Clinical trial of acupuncture for patients with spinal cord injury. *Am J Phys Med Rehabil* 2003; 82(1): 21–27.

12. Honjo H, Kitakoji H, Kawakita K, et al. Acupuncture for urinary incontinence in patients with chronic spinal cord injury. A preliminary report. *Nippon Hinyokika Gakkai Zasshi* 1998; 89: 665–669.

13. Nayak S, Shiflett SC, Schoenberg NE, et al. Is acupuncture effective after treating chronic pain after spinal cord injury? *Arch Phys Med Rehabil* 2001; 82: 1578–1586.

14. Dyson-Hudson TA, Shilett SC, Kirshblum SC, et al. Acupuncture and Trager psychophysical integration in the treatment of wheelchair user's shoulder pain in individuals with spinal cord injury. *Arch Phys Med Rehabil* 2001; 82: 1038–1046.

15. Rapson LM, Wells N, Pepper J, et al. Acupuncture as a promising treatment for below-level central neuropathic pain: a retrospective study. *J Spinal Cord Med* 2003; 26(1): 21–26.

16. Zhu MQ. *Zhu's Scalp Acupuncture*. Hong Kong: 8 Dragons Publishing, 1992.

17. Zhu's Scalp Acupuncture Clinic. Available online at: www.scalpacupuncture. org

18. Cohen K. *The Way of Qigong: The Art and Science of Chinese Energy Healing*. New York: Ballantine Books, 1997.

19. Trieschmann RB. Energy Medicine for Long-Term Disabilities. *Disabil Rehabil* 1999; 21: 269–276.

20. Qigong Database, The Qigong Institute. Available online at: www.qigong institute.org

21. Prasad GC, Khanna RP, Prakash V, et al. Effect of Lajjawanti (*Mimosa pudica linn.*) on regeneration of nerve. *Jur Res Ind Med* 1975; 10(4): 37–44.

22. Maharishi Ayur-Ved Products. Available online at: www.mapi.com

23. Johnston L. Human spinal cord injury: new and emerging approaches to treatment. *Spinal Cord* 2001; 39: 609–613.

3

Laser-Based Therapies

LASER AND LASERPUNCTURE THERAPY

A decade ago when I was director of the Paralyzed Veterans of America's Spinal Cord Research Foundation, a physical therapist called me and related how a man with quadriplegia whom she had been treating with laser therapy had regained considerable function. She asked for assistance in disseminating her function-restoring therapy and findings. Although I provided some advice and referred her to several SCI (spinal cord injury) scientists, in retrospect my assistance was marginal because the system for funding SCI research was designed for mainstream "establishment" efforts of biomedical universities and hospitals and not paradigm-expanding approaches developed by health care practitioners in the field. I regret that I did not do more at the time because I am now convinced that laser-related therapies have considerable potential for treating problems associated with spinal cord injury, including restoring some function.

This book discusses two laser-based therapies in depth. Specifically, this chapter reviews laserpuncture, which has promoted functional recovery in some individuals with SCI; the next chapter discusses a laser therapy for carpal tunnel syndrome and hand spasticity.

Laser Therapy and SCI

Lasers amplify light by producing coherent light beams. Developed in the 1960s, lasers often trigger images of powerful, metal-cutting beams, in part because of movies like *Goldfinger* in which a laser nearly cuts secret agent James Bond in half. In spite of this image, low-energy lasers are finding many therapeutic applications (1). For example, acupuncturists often use lasers instead of needles (2). Overall, lasers represent a noninvasive, painless mechanism for bio-stimulation that does not burn tissue. Scientists speculate that such stimulation improves cellular respiration and function and DNA and RNA repair.

Considerable intriguing research is coming forth, documenting the potential of laser therapy to treat both peripheral nerve and spinal cord injuries. For example, Dr. Semion Rochkind of Tel Aviv, treated 31 patients with severe spinal cord cauda equine injuries (average 3 years postinjury) with laser therapy 6 hours daily for 21 consecutive days. Of these patients, nearly half showed some functional motor improvement (3). Rochkind also examined the effects of embryonic spinal-cord-cell transplantation and laser therapy on recovery after SCI in rats (4). Results indicated that the best recovery of limb function and gait performance, electrophysiological conduction, and histological parameters (indicating implanted tissue growth) occurred after cell implantation and laser radiation. This work is increasingly relevant because several patients who have had neuronal tissue transplanted into their injured cords (5) have augmented this function-restoring surgery with laserpuncture therapy, which is discussed later in this chapter.

Finally, Dr. Kimberly Byrnes et al. of Bethesda, Maryland, demonstrated that laser energy alters gene expression in rats after acute SCI. Their studies indicated that laser energy has an anti-inflammatory effect on the injured cord and may reduce secondary injury, thus providing a possible mechanism by which laser therapy may result in axonal regeneration (6).

Laserpuncture Therapy

As the name implies, laserpuncture combines elements of acupuncture and laser therapy, both of which have shown potential for restoring some function after SCI. Laserpuncture was developed by Albert Bohbot, a French scientist who runs an SCI clinic 120 miles south of Paris (Figure 3-1). Although the use of lasers to stimulate acupuncture points is not new, Bohbot has developed and refined this technology and directed it towards paralysis.

With the support of a technology-transfer grant from the French government and the assistance of scientists at one of France's leading engineering universities, Bohbot developed a sophisticated electronic instrument that substituted an infrared laser light beam

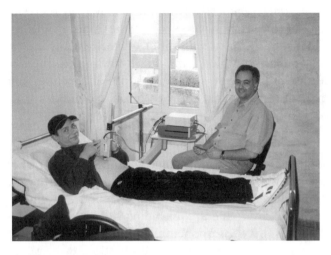

Figure 3-1 Albert Bohbot treating patient with SCI with laserpuncture device. (Photo taken by Laurance Johnston.)

for acupuncture needles. This device specifically emits infrared energy—the part of the electromagnetic spectrum just beyond the limit of visible red light. The power and frequency of this infrared energy can be adjusted to fit the patient's therapeutic needs.

Central to laserpuncture therapy is a network of more than 300 acupuncture points that Bohbot elucidated, based on many years of study, including the examination of ancient Chinese texts. This network relates acupunctural energy meridians to dermatome levels (dermatome matches a specific spinal-cord level with a given area of skin feeling). Bohbot believes that the stimulation of energy through this network restores some function.

Because laserpuncture therapy seems to have restored significant function in many with supposedly complete clinical injuries, Bohbot speculates it is possible to restore some function without intact neurons bridging the spinal injury site. Substituting prevailing biomedical dogma with innovative explanations involving quantum physics and energy medicine, Bohbot believes that there are backup mechanisms to the spinal cord for carrying messages from the brain to the body. He suggests that a signal may be mediated through an electromagnetic energy impulse instead of standard, biochemical conduction through intact neurons using neurotransmitters.

Although my study of esoteric healing indicates that this paradigm-expanding mechanism is theoretically possible, as a conventionally trained biochemist I suggested that improvement might be because of some regeneration or the turning on of residual but dormant neurons that have survived the injury. Scientists now believe that such dormant neurons characterize many injuries clinically classified as "complete" and only a few of these neurons need to be turned on to regain some function. Perhaps laserpuncture is the therapeutic switch that turns them on.

Treatment

Dr. Bohbot has treated many people with SCI, most of whom were at least a year postinjury. Many have regained significant function, although results vary because each injury is unique. Extensive patient experience with laserpuncture, including videos, are posted on Bohbot's Web site (www.laserponcture.net).

Procedurally, in each session the head of the laser device is successively directed toward a series of points on the patient's torso for several minutes each. Based on perceived sensations and any motor or sensory improvement, ensuing sessions may focus on new points and use different energy frequencies. The sessions are augmented with more traditional physical rehabilitation designed to enhance restored function (e.g., walking with leg braces using walkers or parallel bars, riding a stationary bicycle, etc.). Observing Bohbot's patients doing this physical therapy was impressive. Many patients consistently demonstrated regained physical abilities that seemed far beyond what would be possible based on their medical records, a placebo effect, or the physical therapy program by itself.

Bohbot and his colleague Dr. Cécile Jame-Collet studied the effect of this laserpuncture program in 22 individuals with SCI (both paraplegia and quadriplegia) and found that over time, the program increased both thigh and calf circumference (7).

Daniel's Experience

I have talked to many individuals who feel they have accrued substantial benefit from laserpuncture and often routinely traveled great distances to obtain treatment. One of these individuals was Daniel, a member of the Paralyzed Veterans of America. While at the Surface Warfare Officer School in Newport, Rhode Island, Daniel sustained a T-12 injury in a motor vehicle accident 4 months after his 1999 Naval Academy graduation. He noted,

In the last six months working with Albert, I have seen both practical and psychological progress. Gaining the ability to pedal a standard stationary bike and walk in braces has increased my circulation and helped my legs to stay healthy and heal quicker. On top of this physical benefit, such progress has increased my confidence and fed my motivation to work harder. (personal communication, February 10, 2002)

Conclusions

Scientific and extensive anecdotal evidence indicates that laserpuncture, which combines elements of acupuncture and laser therapy, has potential for restoring some function after spinal cord injury.

Additional Readings and Resources

Books

Rochkind S. Laser therapy in the treatment of peripheral nerve and spinal cord injuries. In: Simunovic Z, ed. *Lasers in Medicine and Dentistry: Basic Science and Up-To-Date Clinical Application of Low Energy-Level Laser Therapy*. Rijeka, Croatia: Vitgraf, 2000: 309–318.

Internet

Laserpuncture Clinic: www.laserponcture.net

LASER ACUPUNCTURE FOR CARPAL TUNNEL SYNDROME AND HAND SPASTICITY

Dr. Margaret Naeser, a licensed acupuncturist, research professor at Boston University School of Medicine, and investigator of the Department of Veterans Affairs, has developed an effective alternative therapy for carpal tunnel syndrome (CTS) and spasticity-related hand-flexion problems. Naeser's therapy specifically stimulates acupuncture points of the hand with a low-energy laser beam and a mild electrical current. You can perform this relatively simple and inexpensive therapy at home with some upfront guidance by a licensed acupuncturist. As a mainstream neuroscientist and acupuncturist, Naeser has the cross-disciplinary expertise necessary to integrate Eastern and Western medicine. Because of her unique viewpoint, at a policy-setting 1997 Consensus Development Conference, the National Institutes of Health (NIH) asked her to summarize acupuncture's use in treating central nervous system (CNS) paralysis (8).

Acupuncture

As discussed previously, acupuncture has considerable potential to treat health problems associated with spinal cord injury (SCI). In brief review, acupuncture's philosophy postulates that a life-force energy called qi permeates all living things through channels known as meridians. These meridians are periodically punctuated by acupuncture points, which under traditional theory represent small skin areas that are energy vortexes. As measured by modern scientific measurements, these vortexes correspond to areas of greatly reduced electrical resistance. Stimulating these points through traditional needle insertion, heat, or pressure, or through contemporary energy-emitting devices (e.g., lasers) promotes healthy energy flow. Because most meridians either originate or terminate at the fingertips or tips of the toes, hand and foot disorders seem especially amenable to acupuncture.

Laser Therapy

Naeser's laser acupuncture therapy (9, 10, 11, 12) uses a laser pointer powered by two AAA batteries. It emits a red light beam somewhat similar to a grocery-store checkout scanner and poses no risk unless one stares directly at the beam. Lasers amplify light by producing coherent, single-frequency beams and are characterized by power and wavelength. Their power can vary greatly. For example, 100-watt surgical cutting lasers have 20,000 times the power of the 5-milliwatt laser pointer used in Naeser's program. Because light travels in waves, wavelength refers to the distance measured in nanometers (one billionth of a 39.4-inch meter) between consecutive wave peaks (2). The laser pointer used in Naeser's program emits a 670-nanometer wavelength, corresponding to a red beam of light.

Because low-level lasers represent a noninvasive, painless mechanism for biostimulation, their potential therapeutic applications—including for SCI—have grown greatly over time. When lasers are directed toward acupuncture points, the therapy becomes known as laser acupuncture.

Electrical Stimulation

Naeser's therapy also employs a procedure called microamps transcutaneous electrical nerve stimulation (TENS), using a MicroStim 100 TENS device. In spite of its intimidating name, TENS represents a straightforward procedure, in which mild electric currents are applied to specific skin areas by two circular electrodes that are connected to a pocket-size power pack. TENS devices have a long history of safe use for treating localized pain (although they cannot be used on people who are outfitted with pacemakers).

Carpal Tunnel Syndrome

Carpal tunnel syndrome (CTS) is a painful hand condition caused by compression of the median nerve as it passes through the carpal tunnel from the forearm to the palm. It is aggravated by repetitive motion, including using a wheelchair. Studies indicate that 30% to 73% of manual wheelchair users will experience CTS (13). Conventional CTS treatments include simple hand splinting; steroid injection into the carpel tunnel, which has marginal long-term efficacy; and, surgical release of the impinging ligament.

Although CTS does not generate the visibility of life-threatening disorders, its impact on national health care and worker productivity is immense. For example, surgery is performed in approximately 40% to 45% of CTS cases, with estimates of more than 460,000 procedures performed each year, and a direct medical cost of more than $1.9 billion (3). More than half of all workers afflicted with CTS miss 30 days of work or more per year. Clearly, such statistics warrant the consideration of less expensive, less invasive, and more effective therapeutic alternatives for CTS.

Naeser's approach is supported by substantial scientific evidence, including rigorously designed clinical studies. These studies indicate that approximately 90% of individuals with mild to moderate CTS who are treated with her program three times a week for 4 to 5 weeks by a licensed acupuncturist will have significant enduring relief from CTS pain (9, 10). Naeser believes that these beneficial effects may be mediated through a number of mechanisms, including augmented production of a key energy metabolite called ATP; increased levels of the neurotransmitter serotonin, decreased inflammation, and improved local blood circulation.

Although Naeser's research has focused on CTS, extensive anecdotal observations indicate that the therapy helps spasticity-related hand-flexion difficulties associated with a variety of CNS disorders, such as the fisted or clawed hand. After treatment, the hand relaxes, the fingers can open up more, and existing dexterity may improve. In addition, Naeser's therapy appears to help those who have cramping and spasticity problems in leg and foot muscles.

Treatment

Naeser's straightforward therapy can be carried out readily at home after an acupuncturist has guided the person through it, showing the specific location of the relatively small acupuncture points that are to be targeted by the laser. Readers interested in the therapy should share the protocol (12) with a licensed acupuncturist.

In brief summary, when treating CTS, the MicroStim 100 TENS device's circular lead electrode with blinking red light is attached by means of a sticky patch to the center of the wrist crease, and the grounding pad is attached to the opposite side of the wrist (Figure 3-2). The laser pointer is then directed to fingertip and hand acupuncture points. Because a key acupuncture point is located on the wrist crease, this point is stimulated with the laser before electrode attachment. The 45-minute procedure should be repeated every other day for 5 weeks.

In the case of hand spasticity and flexion problems, the TENS lead electrode is attached to an acupuncture point in the palm and the grounding pad is placed over a point an inch or so above the wrist. Laser stimulation is essentially the same.

Conclusions

This laser-acupuncture therapy is a scientifically proven, highly effective treatment for CTS and may also have considerable potential for treating spasticity-related hand-flexion difficulties.

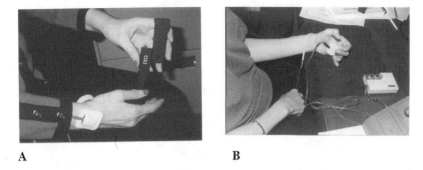

A   B

Figure 3-2 (A and B) The TENS device electrodes are attached to the wrist, and a laser pointer stimulates an acupuncture point on the right hand. A patient with SCI who has spasticity-related hand-flexion difficulties uses an alternative placement for the electrodes.

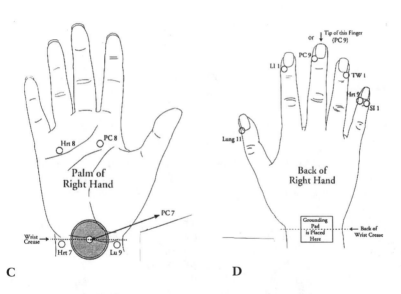

C   D

Figure 3-2 (C and D) (hand diagrams) In the case of carpal tunnel syndrome, these drawings show the location of the placement of the TENS electrodes and the acupuncture points that are to be stimulated by the laser pointer. (Photos and illustrations provided by Dr. Margaret Naeser.)

Additional Reading and Resources

Booklet

Naeser MA, Hahn CK, Lieberman BE. *Naeser Laser Home Treatment Program for the Hand: An Alternative Treatment for Carpal Tunnel Syndrome and Repetitive Strain Injury.* Catasauqua, Penn: American Association of Oriental Medicine, 1997.

Journal Articles

Branco K, Naeser MA. Carpal tunnel syndrome: Clinical outcome After Low-Level Laser Acupuncture, Microamps Transcutaneous Electrical Nerve Stimulation, and Other Alternative Therapies—An Open Protocol Study, *J Altern Complement Med* 1999; 5(1): 5–26.

Liu S. Laser Acupuncture Primer, *California Journal of Oriental Medicine* 2001; 12(1): 23–29.

Naeser MA, Hahn KK, Lieberman BE, et al. Carpal Tunnel Syndrome Pain Treated with Low-Level Laser and Microamps TENS, Controlled Study, *Arch Phys Med Rehabil* 2001; 83: 978–988.

Internet

Naeser M: Laser acupuncture for carpal tunnel syndrome. Available online at: www.acupuncture.com/Acup/Naeser.htm and at www.healingtherapies.info

REFERENCES

1. Naeser MA. Review of second congress, World Association for Laser Therapy meeting (WALT). *J Altern Complement Med* 1999; 5: 177–180.
2. Liu S. Laser acupuncture primer, *California J Oriental Medicine* 2001; 12(1): 23–29.
3. Rochkind, S. Chapter XVI Laser therapy in the treatment of peripheral nerve and spinal cord injuries. In: Simunovic Z (ed). *Lasers in Medicine and Dentistry: Basic Science and Up-To-Date Clinical Application of Low Energy-Level Laser Therapy.* Rijeka, Croatia: Vitgraf, 2000: 309–318.
4. Rochkind S, Shahar A, Amon M, et al. Transplantation of embryonal spinal cord nerve cells cultured on biodegradable microcarriers followed by low power laser irradiation for the treatment of traumatic paraplegia in rats. *Neurol Res* 2002; 24: 355–360.
5. Johnston L. Within the Realm (Olfactory Tissue Transplantation). *Paraplegia News,* 2003; 57(5): 28–32.
6. Byrnes KR, Waynant RW, Ilev IK, et al. Light therapy alters gene expression after acute spinal cord injury. Available online at: www.healingtherapies.info

7. Bohbot A, Jame-Collet C. Restructuring of limb morphology by laserponc-ture® therapy and preliminary research to understand its mechanism of action on muscle activity in patients with spinal cord injury: prospective clinical study of 22 patients with spinal cord injury, who underwent laserponcture® treatment. Available online at: www.healingtherapies.info

8. Naeser MA. Acupuncture in the treatment of paralysis due to central nervous system damage. *J Altern Complement Med* 1996; 2: 211–248.

9. Branco K, Naeser MA. Carpal tunnel syndrome: clinical outcome after low-level laser acupuncture, microamps transcutaneous electrical nerve stimula-tion, and other alternative therapies—an open protocol study. *J Altern Comple-ment Med* 1999; 5(1): 5–26.

10. Naeser MA, Hahn KK, Lieberman BE, et al. Carpal tunnel syndrome pain treated with low-level laser and microamps TENS, controlled study, *Arch Phys Med Rehabil* 2001; 83: 978–988.

11. Naeser MA, Hahn CK, Lieberman BE. *Naeser Laser Home Treatment Program for the Hand: An Alternative Treatment for Carpal Tunnel Syndrome and Repetitive Strain Injury*. Catasauqua, Penn: American Association of Oriental Medi-cine, 1997.

12. Naeser M. Laser acupuncture for carpal tunnel syndrome. Available online at: www.acupuncture.com/Acup/Naeser.htm and at www.healingtherapies.info

13. Cooper R, Bonninger ML, Walking on your hands. *Paraplegia News* 1999; 53(3): 12–16.

4

Natural Health and Vibrational Healing

HOMEOPATHY

Many people with spinal cord injury (SCI) face a life filled with medications. Although clearly providing benefits, these medications often have side effects, which cumulatively over time can have a deleterious health impact. To reduce the SCI medication burden, we need alternatives, such as homeopathy, that augment body defenses.

History

More than 2,000 years ago, Hippocrates, the Father of Western medicine, said: "Through the like, disease is produced, and through the application of the like, disease is cured." Using this philosophy, Dr. Samuel Hahnemann (Figures 4-1, 4-2) developed homeopathy as a medical discipline in the late 18th and early 19th centuries. He discovered that substances that cause symptoms of illness in a healthy person could be used in exceedingly low doses to cure similar symptoms when they result from illness.

For years, homeopathy was very popular. Compared to the relatively backward methodology of 19th century conventional medicine (e.g., blood letting, toxic drugs, etc.), homeopathy was gentle and effective. After Queen Victoria became an advocate, homeopathy became a health-care staple of the English royal family. During various epidemics, the death rate in homeopathic hospitals was much lower than that in conventional hospitals. By the beginning of the 20th century, the United States had 22 homeopathic medical schools and more than 100 homeopathic hospitals. In spite of its popularity,

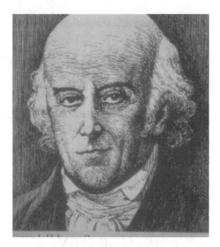

Figure 4-1   Dr. Samuel Hahnemann. (Photo provided by Dana Ullman, Homeopathic Educational Services, Berkeley, CA.)

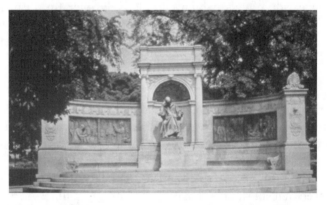

Figure 4-2   The congressionally authorized monument to Dr. Samuel Hahnemann in Washington, DC. (Dana Ullman, Homeopathic Educational Services, Berkeley, CA.)

homeopathy clashed with conventional medicine's objectives and beliefs. Founded in part to fight homeopathy, the American Medical Association (AMA) waged a medical "holy war" against the discipline. For example, AMA members could not be or consult with homeopaths. Because the nonpatentable homeopathic medicines did not generate profits, the AMA found an ally in the drug companies.

Through political machinations, homeopathic schools were stigmatized and regulated out of existence, a process accelerated by conventional medicine's breakthroughs in treating disease. By 1950, no schools and few practitioners remained in the United States.

In recent years, however, homeopathy has enjoyed a renaissance driven by consumers and their desire for health-care options. Currently, homeopathic products are available in most pharmacies. Because of the long history of safe use and small doses of these products, the Food and Drug Administration (FDA) allows selling them without prescription (i.e., they are now over-the-counter drugs). Although most consumers buy the products on their own, there are now several thousand homeopath practitioners in the country, representing a variety of professional disciplines.

Treatment

Conventional medicine focuses on suppressing symptoms or diseases in isolation from the whole person. Because symptoms represent the body's effort to heal itself, symptom-suppressing drugs (e.g., for reducing fever) are counterproductive. In contrast, homeopathy attempts to enhance the body's natural defenses and vital force. Although homeopathy also focuses on symptoms, it does so from a highly individualized, big-picture, mind–body–spirit perspective.

With homeopathy, an individual receives an exceedingly low dose of substance that produces the same symptoms as when the substance is given at toxic levels. For example, toxic doses of arsenic cause diarrhea, weakness, restlessness, and anxiety. When people have the same symptoms due to illness, they can be cured by extremely dilute homeopathic solutions of arsenic. Similarly, ultradilute homeopathic preparations of coffee are used to treat insomnia and restlessness.

For homeopathy to work best, the patient's symptom profile must closely match the toxic symptoms produced when the substance is given at a high dose. These toxic symptoms have been documented for thousands of substances. If the symptom match is close, the treatment can be amazingly effective. The disease name is relatively unimportant. Because ultradiluted homeopathic remedies have few adverse effects, they can be safely used in combination with other medications.

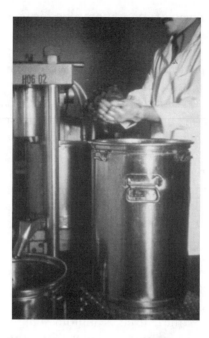

A

Figure 4-3   The preparation of homeopathic medicines: **(A)** Placing the herbs in stainless steel containers to make the mother tinctures. **(B)** The mother tincture is made by macerating the herbs with alcohol for at least three weeks before filtering. **(C)** The process of dilution and shaking takes place in dust-free laboratories. **(D)** The homeopathic solution is dropped onto lactose (milk sugar) globules. **(E)** The final product is stored in plastic or glass containers. (Photo provided by Dana Ullman, Homeopathic Educational Services, Berkeley, CA.)

Homeopathic solutions are prepared by a *potentization* process, in which a mother tincture is serially diluted and shaken. In each cycle, one part of the solution is diluted with nine parts of water and vigorously shaken. The cycle is repeated many times. When a solution has been diluted like this thirty times, it is called 30X. A common 30X preparation represents a 1: 1,000,000,000,000,000, 000,000,000,000,000 (30 zeros) dilution! Although extraordinarily dilute, homeopathic medicines are highly active or potent due to the vigorous shaking between each dilution (Figure 4-3).

It is a paradox that if the symptoms are closely matched, the most dilute solutions are the most powerful. Many homeopathic

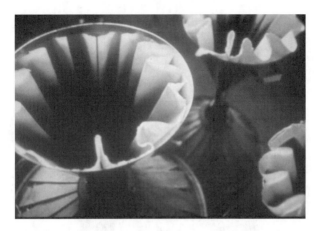

4-3B

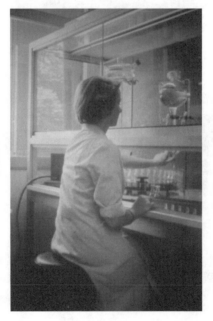

4-3C

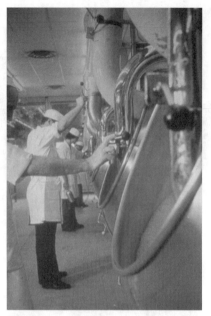

4-3D

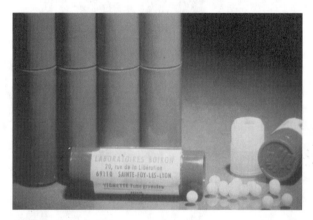

4-3E

products that are sold in pharmacies tend to target a specific disorder (e.g., flu, hay fever, insomnia, etc.) and not the symptoms. As such, lower potencies (ones that are not serially diluted as much) are used, often in combination. This cover-all-the-bases approach may or may not work.

Although based on years of hands-on clinical observations, homeopathy could not be explained by the usual biochemical mechanisms inherent in most physiological processes. Basically, the preparations are so dilute that statistically no molecules remain. Hence, no matter how effective the preparations appeared to be, critics concluded that if nothing was there, the preparations could not work. They dismissed any positive results as being the result of a psychological placebo effect, ignoring that homeopathy worked in unconscious individuals, children, animals, and isolated organs and cells. In recent decades, however, a number of homeopathy preparations have proven to be effective in clinical trials that were rigorously designed to eliminate placebo effects.

Scientific Basis

Electromagnetic Mechanism

Scientists who have started to apply quantum physics and chaos and complexity theory to understanding living systems now believe that homeopathy's effects are mediated indirectly by an electromagnetic mechanism (1). Using sophisticated nuclear magnetic resonance, researchers have shown that homeopathic agents modify water's electromagnetic ultrastructure. This modification is perpetuated through the potentization process and is not diminished but strengthened with increased cycles of dilution and shaking. Even when a homeopathic solution has been filtered to eliminate any remaining molecules, it still possesses activity. Therefore, although the substance itself may have been diluted out, its imprint has not. The snowflake also demonstrates the ability of water to have a "memory." Although each snowflake is unique, it can be melted and then frozen back into its original form.

Consistent with an electromagnetic mechanism, homeopathic effects are destroyed if heated or subjected to magnetic fields. Furthermore, no direct contact with the homeopathic preparation is needed. Specifically, a homeopathic preparation enclosed within a glass vial has been shown to mediate biological effects.

Chaos and Complexity Theory

Researchers explain the translation of homeopathy's subtle electromagnetic energy into physiological effects by using chaos and complexity theory. Basically, under these theories, the flapping of a butterfly's wings can initiate a disturbance that will lead to a hurricane halfway across the world. These theories challenge the scientific reductionism perspective that the whole (e.g., the body) can be understood by breaking down and studying each piece (e.g., organs, hormonal systems, etc.). For example, if a billiard ball is fired against other balls, it is impossible to predict trajectories after a few ricochets, even under ideal circumstances. Nevertheless, scientists attempt to predict outcomes in much more complex systems such as the human body.

With disease, the body's healthy equilibrium has broken down. Due to the complexity of physiological systems, achieving this healthy equilibrium again in any single patient using conventional approaches is difficult. In contrast, homeopathy's strength is based on this complexity. Because a homeopathic remedy is chosen based on an in-depth matching of individual symptoms, it most likely interacts with the same specific, complex systems involved in producing the disease. Through subtle electromagnetic effects, homeopathy cures because it can be likened to affecting the complexity of the forest as a whole and not just a single tree in isolation, as conventional drugs do. It is the uniquely appropriate "butterfly effect" that is needed to shift the body back to health.

Spinal Cord Injury

Because homeopathy has the potential to treat many ailments effectively, it provides a real opportunity for individuals with SCI to reduce their heavy medication burden. Because homeopathy enhances the body's natural defenses, experts recommend that it should be tried first before using conventional medication. However, if you are already using conventional drugs, you can try homeopathic remedies also because they have few side effects.

Homeopathic medicines work best when they closely match the individual's unique symptoms. To some degree, you can do your own matching by consulting consumer guides that are available in bookstores. Even when remedies are based on disease instead of on symptoms, the results can be significant. For example, a popular homeopathic preparation called oscilococcinum (also spelled oscillococcinum) has been proven to be effective in treating flu in double-blind, placebo-controlled clinical trials. Although more hit-or-miss, some homeopathic combination products (i.e., ones containing multiple ingredients) can be effective. For example, they often quickly clear up urinary tract infections.

To obtain the most effective remedies for SCI-associated disorders, you should see a professional homeopath. If this is not feasible, one may benefit from occasionally taking several doses of Hypericum (30X or 30C). Isolated from St. John's wort, Hypericum potentially can help nerve-related injuries, including acute and chronic SCI or SCI-aggravated conditions. Other homeopathic remedies that may be helpful for SCI include Arnica, Cocculus, Natrum sulph, Aurum metallium, Heleborus, Aconitum, and a combination remedy called Traumeel. Homeopaths believe that, ideally, emergency medical technicians should administer homeopathic medicines at accident scenes to minimize injury.

Although little formal research has been carried out in SCI, Dr. Edward Chapman of Boston, Massachusetts, demonstrated that homeopathy significantly lessens the symptoms and improves the functioning of individuals with mild chronic head injury (2). Given such results, it is not unreasonable to expect that homeopathic preparations influence SCI-associated conditions.

Conclusions

By enhancing the body's natural defenses, homeopathy provides a real opportunity for individuals with SCI to reduce their heavy medication burden. Homeopathy is supported by a long history of safe use, many methodologically sound clinical studies, and evolving scientific theory.

Additional Readings and Resources

Books

Bellavite P, Signorini A. *Homeopathy: A Frontier in Medical Science.* Berkeley, Calif.: North Atlantic Books, 1995.

Ullman D. *The Consumer's Guide to Homeopathy: The Definitive Resource for Understanding Homeopathic Medicine and Making it Work for You.* New York: G. P. Putnam, 1995.

Internet

National Center for Homeopathy: www.homeopathic.org
Homeopathic Educational Services: www.homeopathic.com

HERBAL MEDICINE

By helping to maintain health, treat disability-aggravated ailments, and reduce exposure to drug side effects, people with spinal cord injury (SCI) can benefit greatly from herbal medicine.

Years ago, a friend shared with me his herbal health regimen in which he prevented SCI-related urinary tract infections (UTIs) by taking cranberry extract. If he started to get the flu or catch a cold, he took echinacea, and when he was depressed, he consumed St. John's wort.

At that time, my scientific inclinations kept me from embracing such tradition-based remedies, yet my friend was right on target, once again demonstrating why our biomedical experts should listen to health-care consumers with disabilities. Specifically, research now indicates that cranberry prevents UTIs by keeping bacteria from adhering to the bladder lining. Likewise, scientists have determined that echinacea, a Native American medicinal plant, can fight bacterial and viral infections; and St. John's wort, an ancient herbal remedy, is often as effective as antidepressant drugs.

Because of our desire for more natural medicine and remedies, there has been an explosive growth of herbal products, which only a decade ago were relegated to natural food stores and are now displayed prominently in pharmacies and grocery stores. With more than a third of Americans using herbal products, this grassroots, consumer-driven movement is changing the face of the nation's health care.

Although conventional medicine often has botanical connections, herbal medicine is based on a fundamentally different philosophy. Essentially, it relies on natural substances of infinite complexity to address a broad range of bodily experiences. In contrast, pharmaceutically manufactured chemicals target specific disease symptoms and are more likely to produce side effects because they lack the complexity of the natural product that provides buffering for a slower and more diffuse action. Overall, herbal medicine's holistic focus supports wellness by enhancing the body's inherent healing potential. Because it targets the causes of diseases and not merely the symptoms, herbal medicine is more health-promoting rather than disease-killing.

Because of their traditional use over the ages, herbal remedies exist for virtually all ailments, including those that often affect people with SCI. Although proponents and critics may debate the effectiveness of herbal remedies, in many cases when scientists have actually tested them, they work as well as the comparable pharmaceutical drug.

History

Medicinal plants have been always a part of humankind's healing armamentarium and even have been found in Neanderthal burial sites. Ancient cultures, such as the Sumerians and Egyptians in our "cradle of civilization" and the Aztecs and Mayans in the Western Hemisphere, relied on plants for medicines. Herbal medicine is the cornerstone of age-old, Eastern healing disciplines that live on today. Some of these include Traditional Chinese Medicine and India's Ayurvedic medicine, which both have become increasingly popular recently in the West.

Indigenous healing traditions also emphasized medicinal plants, and many became incorporated into Western medicine. For example, more than 200 Native American herbal medicines have been listed at one time in the U.S. Pharmacopoeia, an official compendium of drugs and medicines. Herbal medicine also laid the foundation for Western medicine. The Ancient Greeks—including Hippocrates, the Father of Medicine—and in turn the Romans relied extensively on herbal remedies. Through the Dark Ages, herbal knowledge was preserved by Islamic cultures and by village women, many of whom were burned at the stake as witches because of their healing talents. The discovery of numerous New World medicinal plants stimulated renewed interest in herbal remedies, and as a result, by the mid-1800s most Western medicines were plant derived. The interest in herbal medicine subsided, however, as a schism began to grow between botany and medicine. We started to lose our connection to nature as society became more industrialized, and as pharmaceutical companies began to chemically synthesize patentable, money-making drugs. As modern medicine evolved around pharmaceutical concepts, it neglected herbal remedies. Currently, U.S. physicians obtain most of their information on medicines from the pharmaceutical industry, a giant economic force.

Today's World

Once again, the tide is turning. Many doctors are revisiting herbal remedies in response to consumer interest. And, as consumers themselves, 40% of family physicians also use them. In addition, herbal alternatives increasingly are being used to control soaring healthcare costs. For example, one Oklahoma HMO prescribes St. John's wort instead of Prozac because the herb appears to be just as effective yet is much cheaper (3). Although we may think our pharmaceutically based medical practices are the norm for the world, this is not true. Most of the world's population rely on herbal remedies because they cannot afford Western drugs. Even in many wealthy nations, herbal remedies are being reintegrated into mainstream medicine (4). For example, in Germany and France, millions of herbal prescriptions are written each year, ginkgo biloba is prescribed more often than any pharmaceutical, and 30% to 40% of all doctors rely on herbal remedies as their primary medications.

Regulatory Philosophy

Although Americans have ready access to herbal remedies, few are used officially as medicines. To protect consumer access to these remedies from FDA regulatory zeal, Congress in 1994 adopted legislation classifying them as dietary supplements, provided they claim only to affect the body's structure and function. However, if an herbal product claims it can treat or cure an ailment, it would then be considered a drug, and hence subjected to the arduous, expensive FDA drug-regulatory process. Because herbs cannot be patented, no financial incentives exist for profit-making companies to seek such a drug designation. Under this regulatory approach, semantics become important. For example, if an herbal product claims to cure UTIs instead of just promoting urinary tract health, it is considered a drug.

Single Versus Multicomponent Remedies

More than 30% of modern medicine's drugs have botanical origins. For example, willow tree bark contains salicylic acid, aspirin's active agent; cinchona bark has malaria-fighting quinine; foxglove digitalis treats congestive heart failure; rosy periwinkle has leukemia-fighting chemicals; and the evergreen ephedra is commonly used in decongestants. Even lifesaving penicillin, which revolutionized SCI health care, was isolated from molds that were used as folk remedies. Given such a botanical basis, why does modern medicine struggle so much with herbal remedies? After all, pharmaceuticals *and* herbs mediate their action through physiologically active molecules. Part of the answer is that the acceptance of herbal healing would challenge modern medicine's belief that it is a scientifically driven instead of an empirically based discipline.

Specifically, modern medicine's use of drugs is based on rigorously designed clinical trials, whereas herbal use is based on centuries of experience. Because the pharmaceutical approach focuses on only one molecularly defined drug, scientists can evaluate cause and effect more readily, determine mechanisms of action, and define appropriate dosing. Such assessments are difficult for complex herbal remedies that possess a multitude of biologically active components. As such, scientists prefer initially to isolate a remedy's active agents, believing that overall activity will be the sum of the component parts. This reductionistic view, however, is rarely true because the plant components act more in concert than individually to create the overall healing effect. In many cases, scientists have been disappointed to discover that the isolated agent had less activity than the crude herb.

Standardization

Biological activity can vary substantially between herbal preparations. For example, it depends on the parts harvested (i.e., leaves, roots, flowers, stems), plant maturity, soil and environmental conditions, and appropriate preparation and storage. It is truly a healing art, which at times has confounded ethnobiologists, who have been provided exciting new medicinal plants by shamanic healers but who could not later duplicate their initial success when they harvested the plants themselves. The variability in activity among supposedly comparable products is a major criticism of herbal medicine and inhibits its acceptance by doctors, who understandably are more confident prescribing medicines at clearly defined doses. Some herbal products have been prepared without good quality control and lack standardization. There have been cases, independent of price or brand name, of products that contain little biologically active agent.

Although many companies now attempt to standardize their products, this process can be controversial also. For example, if a given herbal preparation lacks sufficient activity, it may be spiked with additional active ingredients. Such spiking creates a chemical imbalance that diminishes the natural synergy of plant components, violating herbal medicine's supposed philosophical foundation.

Safety

When prepared with good quality control, most herbal remedies are gentle and unlikely to cause serious side effects. Nevertheless, because like drugs they contain physiologically active agents, some side effects can occur. In practice, however, the most common are allergic reactions, throat irritations, gastrointestinal upsets, and headaches. When more serious side effects do occur, the medical establishment frequently touts that as a reason for people to stay away from herbal remedies. This is a double standard because the documented incidence of serious reactions to herbal remedies is much less than that of reactions to pharmaceuticals. Specifically, it has been estimated that herbal remedies cause 50 to 100 deaths annually. In comparison, studies suggest that adverse reactions to hospital-administered drugs cause 105,000 deaths annually, making it the country's 4th to 6th leading cause of death (5). Given such statistics, people with SCI, who often face a heavy medication burden, may be better off using herbal medicine for routine ailments and saving the heavy pharmaceutical artillery for the more serious conditions.

Herbal Applications

By helping to maintain health, treat SCI-aggravated ailments, and reduce exposure to drug side effects, people with SCI can benefit greatly from herbal medicine. Furthermore, the use of infection-fighting herbal remedies that enhance the body's inherent healing potential will help preserve the effectiveness of lifesaving antibiotics over time.

Many herbs support and nourish the nervous system. For example, as discussed elsewhere in this book, the Ayurvedic herb *Mimosa pudica* (sensitive plant) has been shown to promote neuronal regeneration in animal studies and may benefit some people with SCI as indicated by a small pilot study carried out by the author (6). In addition, Feather Jones, director of the Rocky Mountain Center for Botanical Studies in Boulder, Colorado, has suggested that several other nerve-nourishing herbs potentially may help in spinal cord dysfunction. For example, she has indicated that a fresh plant extract of skullcap (a member of the mint family) reduces nerve inflammation; a tincture of milky oats (immature oat seeds) can rebuild the neuronal myelin sheath that is often damaged in both multiple sclerosis and SCI; an external liniment of cow parsnip, (a common weed that is a member of the parsley family) is a traditional Southwestern Hispanic remedy for treating injured nerves and stimulating regeneration. External application of St. John's wort can treat neural inflammation, and hawthorn helps to hold collagen fibers in place along the spinal cord.

Given such effects, the potential for these remedies to treat people in the SCI acute phase seems intriguing and deserving of further research.

Herbal Favorites

The following is a sampling of some of the more popular herbal remedies:

Bilberry enhances eye health, including improving night vision and preventing cataracts, macular degeneration, and glaucoma.

Cranberry prevents urinary tract infections.

Echinacea (purple coneflower) fights cold, flu, urinary tract and other infections by stimulating the immune system (Figure 4-4). (Because multiple sclerosis appears to be an autoimmune disease, some believe that echinacea should not be used when one has multiple sclerosis.)

Garlic fights bacterial, viral, and parasitic infections, reduces high blood pressure, lowers cholesterol, prevents atherosclerosis, and is associated with lower cancer rates.

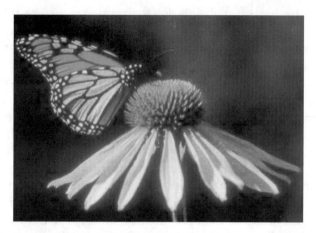

Figure 4-4 Echinacea, a Native-American herb, can fight bacterial and viral infections. (Photo provided by Michael Moore.)

Ginger treats digestive disorders such as nausea and vomiting, motion sickness; and inhibits immune-system components that promote inflammation in rheumatoid arthritis.

Ginko biloba increases blood circulation, especially in the brain, enhancing memory and mental alertness.

Ginseng has stimulant properties useful for chronic fatigue, convalescence, lethargy, depression, and chronic infections due to immune weakness. Ginseng can help diabetics by lowering blood sugar.

Hawthorn strengthens the heart and prevents heart disease. It reduces blood pressure, angina attacks, atherosclerosis, and treats congestive heart failure.

Kava treats anxiety, mild depression, and insomnia.

Saw palmetto eases symptoms associated with prostate inflammation or enlargement.

St. John's wort treats depression and insomnia.

Valerian's sedative properties promote sleep.

Conclusions

Herbal and conventional medicine are part of a healing spectrum, in which each has something positive, yet different, to offer. Although conventional medicine's high-technology approaches are especially useful in treating acute disease and in emergency care, by supporting wellness, herbal medicine is more suitable for dealing with the chronic ailments that are increasingly affecting modern society. Because herbal medicine addresses an important health-care need, its continued integration into the mainstream should benefit everyone, including people with SCI.

Additional Readings and Resources

Books

Balch PA. *Prescription for Herbal Healing.* New York: Penguin Putnam, 2002.
Hobbs C. *Herbal Remedies for Dummies.* Foster City, Calif.: IDG Books Worldwide, 1998.
Keville K. *Herbs for Health and Healing.* New York: Berkley Books, 1996.
Murray MT. *The Healing Power of Herbs.* Rocklin, Calif.: Prima Publishing, 1995.
Swerdlow JL. *Nature's Medicine—Plants that Heal.* Washington, DC: National Geographic, 2000.

AROMATHERAPY AND ESSENTIAL OILS

Aromatherapy, or essential-oil therapy, is a natural, gentle treatment that can be used as an adjunct and sometimes as an alternative to the many conventional pharmaceutical medications that people with spinal cord injury (SCI) frequently rely upon. By expanding the healing armamentarium available to us, these oils have the potential to reduce our reliance on these pharmaceuticals and exposure to their side effects.

Smells can trigger vivid memories, involving sights, sounds, and emotional impressions of events in our distant past. With me, for example, a whiff of oatmeal cookies evokes childhood memories of my grandmother baking her culinary morsels of affection in a wood stove in her northern Minnesota kitchen. In addition to such memories, smells can initiate a cascade of physiological responses that affect our entire body and mental outlook.

These responses form the basis for an ancient healing tradition now called aromatherapy, a term coined by Rene Gatfosee, a French perfume-industry chemist. Gatfosee worked with volatile plant essential oils for making fragrances until one day when he had an explosion in his lab and was badly burned. He plunged his arm into the nearest vat of liquid, which happened to be lavender. To his amazement, the pain stopped immediately, and no blistering or scarring occurred. As a result, he changed his focus completely to the medicinal effects of these oils.

Aromatherapy can be confusing to the layperson. As "natural" products have become more popular and aromatherapy a buzzword, commercial interests began to slap the term "aromatherapy" on everything that had a fragrance. A layperson tends to think, "Aromatherapy is everything that stinks." Well, you cannot have aromatherapy without essential oils, but you can have essential oils without its being aromatherapy. The difference is in the application and intent. Aromatherapy is the use of essential oils with the goal of causing a positive change physically, emotionally, mentally, or spiritually. For example, many shampoos contain essential oils, but that is not aromatherapy. True aromatherapy would be when you choose particular essential oils to add to your shampoo for a specific intent, for example, to encourage hair growth, fight a specific physiological condition of the scalp, help clarify the mind, encourage memory, and center and relax yourself before a big day.

Ancient Origins

Alchemists labeled aromatic plant oils *essential* because they believed the fragrances reflected the plant's true inner nature. Throughout history, the oils have been used for healing and are still key elements of many of the world's non-Western healing traditions. For example, India's Ayurvedic healing tradition routinely uses essential-oil fragrances to obtain the right *doshic* balance needed for good health. Indian sages believed fragrances affected human consciousness, and so encouraged rituals of worship that incorporated flowers. To this day, flowers are an integral part of daily worship and activity throughout India. Everywhere you go, you will see people making flower garlands, which are used daily to adorn household, village, and field and temple shrines. The garlands are blessed at temple and then given back to the worshipper, who wears it throughout the day. It is believed the constant exposure to these highly evolved fragrances refines and elevates consciousness.

Ancient Egyptians really are to be credited for the most complex uses of the oils. To Egyptians, fragrance was of the utmost importance as their goal was divinity. Bathing, anointing, and using fragrances would lead to holiness. In death, people must smell of this holiness in order to be acceptable to the gods, and therefore the sacred oils that corresponded to each organ would be used on the body after death. This ancient wisdom receded because of history, politics, and religion. After Alexander the Great conquered Egypt, the victors wanted all the essential-oil formulas, especially aphrodisiacs and those that gave power over others. Because the Greeks had no spirituality goal, the Egyptian priests gave them incomplete formulas with ingredients missing. The Romans took the abuse of oils to great heights, having a fortune in oils go through their fountains, and using them in orgies of food and drink, and so forth. Christian priests condemned this lasciviousness and forbade the use of essential oils. The schism began between holistic, consciousness-influencing usage and specific medical and cosmetic applications of essential oils.

Modern Times

In recent years as natural health-care alternatives have been sought out, aromatherapy has seen a remarkable renaissance. In Europe, it is considered an effective treatment that is increasingly being integrated with conventional medicine and reimbursed by insurance companies.

Many investigations demonstrate aromatherapy's effectiveness, including double-blind studies designed to eliminate the psychological placebo effect. Unfortunately, the U.S. medical establishment has not accessed many of the studies because they have been published in other languages or represent proprietary information of the flavor and fragrance industry. Yet, studies have yielded many interesting findings. For example, keypunch-operator errors were cut in half after lemon scent was piped through the ventilation system. As a result, Japanese corporations use various scents to increase worker performance. In another example, New York subway passengers became less aggressive when the cars were scented with pleasant food aromas. And finally, eucalyptus oil keeps truck drivers as alert as caffeine does.

Extraction Isolation

Essential oils are routinely extracted from plants by using steam distillation (Figure 4-5). As the steam percolates through the plant material, it pulls off volatile oils, which are then condensed. Huge quantities of raw plant material are often needed to obtain a small amount of oil. In the case of rose oil, it takes 2,000 pounds of petals to produce one pound of oil. Essential oils are highly concentrated. For example, the chemicals in one drop of oil are equivalent to thirty cups of a tea prepared from plant material. These oils are also highly complex, containing from 100 to 400 different chemical compounds in one oil, giving a wide range of seemingly improbable properties within the same oil.

Because of the cost of making essential oils, most commercial product fragrances are chemically synthesized. Although such synthetics may superficially smell like the real thing, synthetics do not work in the body in the same way, are not readily eliminated, and tend to provoke more allergic reactions.

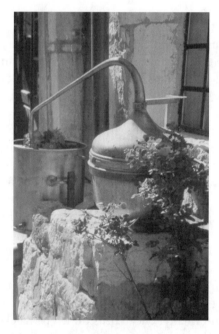

Figure 4-5   Essential oils are routinely extracted from plants using steam distillation. (Photo provided by Pamela Parsons.)

How Essential Oils Enter the Body

Although numerous ways exist to administer essential oils, the most common are through the nose and the skin.

Nose

Volatile oils can affect the body through the highly sensitive *olfactory system*. When cells located in the upper part of the nose capture odor molecules, signals go to the brain's limbic region, a primitive portion of the brain. This region controls the body's basic survival functions, in part by influencing key hormone-secreting glands that affect the entire body. Hence, a smell can quickly influence your entire body. These actions are below the threshold of consciousness. Hence, the most important functions necessary to our survival are powerfully affected by smell—and we don't even know it. You don't need to be aware of the smell at all to be affected. The same is true for odors that bring disharmony and imbalance. For example, the pheromones of fear and violence can trigger the same in another, increasing violence. You can inhale essential oils in many ways: Several drops can be placed in bath water, in a nearby bowl of warm water, in a humidifier or on a lightbulb, in the melted wax surrounding a lit candle, or on a handkerchief. You can also purchase inexpensive diffusion devices.

Skin

Oils absorbed through skin pores and hair follicles enter bloodstream capillaries and circulate throughout the body. Because you smell the fragrances as the oil is rubbed on your skin, it is difficult to separate effects resulting from topical administration from inhalation. Unlike many chemicals or drugs, essential oils do not accumulate and are quickly excreted from the body. Furthermore, unlike medications that must be swallowed and systemically absorbed, locally applied essential oils bypass the stomach and liver and therefore are not compromised by metabolic alteration. They go directly to the spot where they are needed the most (e.g., sore muscle, bruise, etc.). Because essential oils are highly concentrated, they are usually diluted before being applied to the skin through oil-based mixtures, such as salves, creams, or lotions; alcohol- or water-based tinctures; or with a compress (a water-soaked cloth).

Applications

In *psychoaromatherapy*, essential oils are used either to stimulate or to relax the brain. Some oils can have calming and tranquilizing effects; others are energizing and can help relieve depression. These oils can relief stress and anxiety and promote a general feeling of well being. In *therapeutic aromatherapy*, essential oils treat medical conditions. For example, they can fight infections, promote wound healing, reduce inflammation, affect hormonal levels, stimulate the immune system, heat the skin in a liniment, promote blood circulation and digestion, and lessen sinus or lung congestion. *Aesthetic aromatherapy* focuses on beauty issues such as hair and skin care.

Aromatherapy can treat many ailments, including those frequently associated with SCI. For example, *Aromatic Thymes* magazine published a case study in which aromatherapy was used to enhance the health of a quadriplegic in the acute injury phase (7). Specifically, essential oils were used to prevent respiratory infections, promote mucus clearing, fight depression, and promote sleep. Although a few applications are listed below, readers are encouraged to look at the resource references for particular remedies relevant to their needs.

Specific Aromatherapy Applications

Pain

Often applied through massage oils, lotions, liniments, or compresses, essential oils reduce pain by different mechanisms:

Numbing: Some oils—such as clove bud, frankincense, chamomile, lavender, and lemongrass—dull pain by numbing nerve endings.

Anti-inflammatory: Oils such as chamomile, geranium, juniper, lavender, marjoram, myrrh, rose, and tea tree diminish pain through anti-inflammatory actions.

Heat: Some oils—for example, bay laurel, bay rum, black pepper, cinnamon, clove bud, ginger, juniper, peppermint, and thyme—relieve pain by producing heat and increasing circulation.

Brain: Some oils—such as frankincense, ginger, and lemongrass—interfere with the brain's processing of pain signals.

Neurotransmitters: Oils such as birch (containing aspirin-like compounds), cayenne, and ginger hinder the production of neurotransmitters that carry pain messages from nerve endings to the central nervous system.

Relaxation: Using chamomile, clary sage, lavender, lemon, lemon eucalyptus, lemon verbena, marjoram, melissa (lemon balm), myrtle, and petitgrain (a citrus-related plant) may help relieve pain through relaxation.

Insomnia

Sleep-promoting oils—including bergamot, chamomile, clary sage, frankincense, geranium, lavender, melissa, mandarin, neroli (orange blossom), rose, sandalwood, and tangerine—can be inhaled, rubbed on the skin with massage oil or lotion, or used in bath water.

Headaches

When inhaled, a variety of oils—including lavender, melissa, peppermint, basil, chamomile, lemongrass and marjoram—can relieve headaches of different origins.

Stress

Some oils—including bergamot, chamomile, lavender, lemon, melissa, marjoram, neroli, petitgrain, rose, sandalwood, and valerian—relieve stress (even slowing brain waves).

Depression

Antidepressant qualities are found in some oils such as angelica, bergamot, cardamom, chamomile, cinnamon, clary sage, clove, cypress, lavender, lemon verbena, lemon, melissa, orange, neroli, petitgrain, rose, and ylang-ylang (a tropical Asian tree).

Stimulation

Many oils will stimulate and keep you alert: angelica, basil, benzoin (from a tree of Southeast Asia), black pepper, cardamom, cinnamon, clove, cypress, ginger, jasmine, peppermint, rosemary, and sage.

High Blood Pressure

Oils have been shown to lower blood pressure, including neroli, orange, melissa, tangerine, rose, ylang-ylang, geranium, and clary sage.

Bacterial Infections

Oils isolated from bay laurel, cinnamon, clove bud, garlic, oregano, savory, and thyme are powerful antibacterial agents (albeit potential skin irritants). More gentle antibacterial oils include bay rum, benzoin, cardamom, eucalyptus, frankincense, geranium lavender, lemon, lemongrass, marjoram, myrrh, myrtle, pine rose, sage, and tea tree. These oils can treat infections of the skin, bladder, bowel, ear, gums, sinus, skin, and throat. The nature of the infection will determine whether the oils are inhaled or rubbed on the skin. Urinary tract infections (UTIs) can be treated with baths, sitz baths, and massages using certain essential oils. For example, a massage oil containing niaouli, cajeput (both a type of tea tree oil) or sandalwood can be rubbed into the abdomen and kidney region of the lower back. Cuts and wounds can be treated with sprays or salves that contain essential oils isolated from eucalyptus, lavender, lemon, thyme, marjoram, rosemary, tea tree, or basil.

Viral Infections

Often used as ingredients in cough drops and cold and flu medications, many oils also have antiviral properties. These oils include bay, bergamot, black pepper, cardamom, cinnamon bark, clove bud, eucalyptus, garlic, geranium, holy basil, juniper, lavender, melissa, lemongrass, lemon, marjoram, myrrh, oregano, rose, rosemary sage, tea tree, and thyme.

Conclusions

Aromatherapy or essential-oil therapy is a natural, gentle treatment that expands the SCI healing armamentarium, thereby reducing reliance on pharmaceuticals that often carry many side effects. Get well with smell!

Acknowledgment

The assistance of Pamela Parsons, founder and former publisher of *Aromatic Thymes* magazine, is greatly appreciated.

Additional Readings and Resources

Books

Cooksley VG. *Aromatherapy: A Lifetime Guide to Healing with Essential Oils.* Paramus, NJ: Prentice-Hall, 1996.
Keville K. *Aromatherapy for Dummies.* Foster City, Calif.: IDG Books Worldwide, 1999.
Masline SR, Close B. *Aromatherapy: The A–Z Guide to Healing with Essential Oils.* New York: Dell Publishing, 1998.

FLOWER ESSENCES

Unlike herbal remedies or aromatherapy's essential oils, flower essences mediate their healing without pharmacologically active molecules. Representing a higher vibrational octave of the plant's herbal or molecular properties, flower essences energetically restore balance on physical, emotional, and spiritual levels. Because all disability has many nonphysical mental and spiritual components, flower essences greatly expand the SCI healing spectrum.

No biologically active molecules essentially exist in a flower-essence solution. Therefore, it is difficult for biomedical professionals and scientists—who are trained to explain biological phenomena through molecular interactions (e.g., neurotransmitter interacting with a receptor on the neuronal cell surface)—to understand how molecule-free essences can work. Understanding requires that we revisit a concept inherent to most ancient and indigenous healing traditions: that the body's physiology and biochemistry are a function of our being, first and foremost, beings of energy.

Flower Essences = Energy Medicine

As discussed elsewhere in this book, the alternative-medicine practitioners believe that our attitudes and emotions are transformed into our biochemistry and physiology through subtle electromagnetic fields that permeate and surround our bodies. It is through these fields that flower essences are thought to exert their mind–body–spirit healing effects. Specifically, the flower's electromagnetic patterns that have been released into the solution interact with the body's electromagnetic fields, restoring energetic balance and in turn physical health. Flower essences' subtle energetic influences have been compared, for example, to the uplifting effects we experience listening to inspirational music or seeing majestic views. Through what scientists call *psychoneuroimmunological* mechanisms, these feelings manifest into beneficial and measurable physical changes.

Bach to Basics

Flower-essence healing was influenced by the thinking of Paracelsus (1493–1541), one of history's most prominent physicians, and the well-known German poet and nature scientist Johann Wolfgang von Goethe (1749–1832). Paracelsus believed what is called the "doctrine of signatures," namely, that plants' physical forms revealed their therapeutic potential in how they corresponded to human anatomy. Goethe's holistic approach to natural science, perhaps because of his poetic insight, reflected the soulfulness of and connection to nature, an approach that contrasted to the prevailing scientific method of reductionistic analysis.

Although a part of ancient healing traditions, English physician Edward Bach (1886–1936) catalyzed the modern reemergence of flower essences. A conventionally trained physician, Bach specialized in bacteriology and vaccine development. He later shifted to homeopathy, philosophically a close relative to flower essences. In 1930, Bach quit his practice and devoted the last six years of his life to developing his thirty-eight well-known flower essences. Bach's holistic healing view was emphasized in his writings. For example, in *Heal Thyself,* (8) he says:

> Disease is in essence the result of a conflict between soul and mind and will never be eradicated except by spiritual and mental effort. . . . No effort directed to the body alone can do more than superficially repair damage and in this is no cure since the cause is

still operative and may at any moment again demonstrate its presence in another form. (p. 10)

Because each plant has the potential to be transformed into a unique healing essence, many new flower essences have been developed in response to the therapy's popularity.

Preparation

Flower essences are prepared by placing flower petals—the plant part believed to have the most life force—into a glass bowl filled with water. The bowl is placed under sunlight, which melds the flower's energetic imprint into the water. Although nothing physical gets transferred, using highly specialized photographic procedures, the flower's energy imprint has been observed on the solution after removing the flowers. This sun infusion is called the *mother tincture*, which in turn is often diluted and preserved with brandy. You commonly administer essences by placing several drops under the tongue.

Selecting Flower Essences

Determining an essence's healing properties is an intuitive, observational process—so to speak, a communion with nature that reflects Paracelsus' statement "If you wish to know the book of nature, you must walk its pages with your feet." Patiently observing the plant and perceiving its manifold characteristics results in insights that are translated into healing attributes. These attributes are usually defined at the emotional and mental level and often verified through user feedback.

Because of the plethora of available essences, selecting the right ones can be difficult. Traditionally, you would attempt to identify your underlying, health-affecting emotional and mental issues and then match these to essence healing attributes as listed in various resources or repertories. For example, the Bach sweet chestnut, gorse, wild oat, and wild rose essences are indicated for depression or despair-related health issues (8).

Because of the difficulty in accurately identifying health-affecting core issues, a muscle-testing procedure called *kinesiology* can be used to select essences. Such kinesiology is a commonly used in numerous alternative healing traditions to determine the appropriateness of a specific therapeutic approach for a unique individual. Basically, in the case of essences, you hold an essence in one hand while another person attempts to force down gently the opposite outstretched arm. If the remedy energetically resonates with you, it will subconsciously increase your strength, and you will resist more force than with an unneeded remedy. Machelle Small Wright, creator of Perelandra flower essences, has simplified this procedure by developing a self-test involving finger strength, as well as alternative procedures when disability inhibits finger testing (9). Although kinesiology theoretically eliminates the need to identify often complex and vague underlying mental and emotional health determinants, it requires some skill gained through experience. Without the skill, flower-essence selection can be a hit-or-miss process.

Fortunately, several combination remedies are available that provide wide-spectrum healing protection. For example, the Bach Rescue Remedy, composed of five key flower essences, exerts a stabilizing effect for many physical and mental stresses. This product alone represents 43% of the U.S. flower-essence market. Based on nearly 70 years of case studies, the remedy is considered the emergency first-aid of flower essences because it prevents the disintegration of our energy system after physical or emotional trauma, thereby promoting physical recovery. This is the remedy to be used immediately after a SCI.

Another popular combination remedy is the Flower Essence Society's Yarrow Special Formula. Developed in response to the 1986 Chernobyl nuclear plant disaster, the remedy protects your energy field's integrity from harmful environmental influences, especially from all types of unnatural radiation that now ubiquitously affects modern society (e.g., dental x-rays, airport-detection devices, computer monitors, cellular phones, etc.).

Flower-Essence Science

Concepts of soul healing and molecule-independent energy mechanisms are troublesome for most scientists. Nevertheless, Dr. Jeffrey Cram, a clinical research psychologist with extensive scientific credentials, has shown in several controlled studies that flower essences can, indeed, exert measurable physiological effects (10, 11). Specifically, Cram's studies show that the aforementioned combination remedies can reduce the stress response induced by various situations as measured by skin temperature and conductance and various elec-trophysiological parameters, such as brain waves and muscle elec-trical activity. Intriguingly, the flower-essence responses were espe-cially notable at locations corresponding to specific *chakra* sites, which according to ancient wisdom are the points in which the flow of life-force pranic energy into the body is the greatest. Cram also examined the use of flower essences to treat depression. Preliminary results indicated that the essences have comparable effectiveness to many antidepressant drugs.

Spinal Cord Injury

Flower essences expand the healing spectrum available to people with SCI, enhancing health and wellness and therefore potentially reducing the side effects associated with a heavy medication burden. Unfortunately, little focus has been placed on the therapy's healing potential uniquely relevant to SCI.

Alternative healers believe that SCI profoundly disturbs the body's energetic patterns, inhibiting physiological healing. With this view, any therapy that stabilizes these patterns has healing potential. Wright speculates that flower essences are one of these therapies: "I would love to get essences in on spinal cord injuries," she states. "This is the thing I think that would take spinal cord injury right over the top because now you've got an electrical pattern that's going to be addressing the very base of your electrical opera-tion; the nerve center. And I think when you're talking about regen-eration and you put that electrical system on, it will regenerate." (12)

The book *Flower Essences and Vibrational Healing* (13) alludes to several essences that may have relevance to spinal cord dysfunction. For example, comfrey and khat (native to Africa) essences are indicated as potentially beneficial for rejuvenating or regenerating damaged neurological tissue. The poppy and chamo-mile essences supposedly enhance the body's assimilation of gold, the lack of which according to the medical intuitive Edgar Cayce is responsible for causing or aggravating many neurological disorders, including SCI.

Conclusions

Because SCI has so many nonphysical aspects at the deepest soul level, the mind–body–spirit approach of flower essences expands our healing spectrum beyond therapies directed to the mere physical. Although the underlying philosophy of flower essences until recently has fallen beyond the pale of orthodox scientific thinking, if there is one scientific truth it is that today's cutting-edge insights are often tomorrow's anachronisms. As Paracelsus stated, "That which is looked upon by one generation as the apex of human knowledge is often considered an absurdity by the next, and that which is regarded as a superstition in one century, may form the basis of science for the following one."

Additional Readings and Resources

Books

Bach Flower Remedies. The Unique Healing Treatment: Why it Works and How to Benefit from its 38 Powerful Essences. New Canaan, CT: Keats Publishing, 1997.

Devi L. *The Essential Flower Essence Handbook*. Carlsbad, Calif.: Hay House, 1996.

Gerber R. *Vibrational Medicine for the 21st Century*. New York: HarperCollins, 2000.

Gurudas. *Flower Essences and Vibrational Healing*. San Rafael, Calif.: Cassandra Press, 1989.

Kaminski P, Katz R. *Flower Essence Repertory: A Comprehensive Guide to North American and English Flower Essences for Emotional and Spiritual Well-Being*. Nevada City, Calif.: The Flower Essence Society, 1996.

Scheffer M. *Bach Flower Therapy: Theory & Practice*. Rochester, Vt.: Healing Arts Press, 1988.

Wright MS. *Flower Essences: Reordering Our Understanding and Approach to Illness and Health*. Warrenton, Va.: Perelandra, 1988.

Vlamis G. *Bach Flower Remedies to the Rescue*. Rochester, Vt.: Healing Arts Press, 1990.

Videos and Audiotapes

Wright MS. *The Human Electrical System and Flower Essences* [videotape]. Warrenton, Va.: Perelandra, 1996.

Wright MS. *Flower Essences II Workshop: Perelandra Tape Series 6* [audiotape]. Warrenton, VA: Perelandra, 1993.

Internet

Flower Essence Society: www.flowersociety.org

Nelson Bach USA Ltd.: www.nelsonbach.com

Pegasus Flower Essence Products: www.pegasusproducts.com

Perelandra Center for Nature Research: www.perelandra-ltd.com

EDGAR CAYCE'S VISION: THE GOLDEN TOUCH

Every man takes the limits of his own field of vision for the limits of the world.

—Arthur Schopenhauer

This book has sought out nontraditional viewpoints that provide a different "vision for the limits of the world," and in turn what may be possible for spinal cord injury (SCI). Although this search often has gone beyond the banks of mainstream medicine, it has been rarely based on a source as unusual as Edgar Cayce (Figure 4-6), America's most famous medical intuitive and psychic. Because Cayce's uncanny insights have had astonishing validity for many ailments and disorders, we should set aside the mystique surrounding him and attempt to look with an open mind at what he had to say about spinal cord dysfunction.

History has taught us that many scientific and medical breakthroughs are based on insights from nontraditional sources, ranging from shamanic medicine men to folk remedies to, in this case, the medical intuitive. Our wisdom resides not so much in accepting or

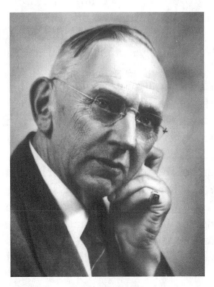

Figure 4-6   Photo of Edgar Cayce. (Photo provided by Association of Research and Enlightenment, Virginia Beach, VA.)

rejecting these sources but in listening to what they have to say. In the case of intuitive insights, in fact, many famous scientists have acknowledged that their discoveries were based on "out-of-the-blue" epiphanies, although rarely was it of the magnitude demonstrated by Cayce, a person with no medical or scientific training.

Cayce's Background

Cayce was born in 1877 in rural Kentucky. He had relatively limited formal education, although what he did receive was augmented by his enviable ability to be able to master a topic by sleeping with his head resting on his textbook. While reading the bible and praying in the woods when he was 13, Cayce claimed that an angel-like being visited him and said that his prayers about wanting to heal the sick had been answered. Indeed, the first person Cayce healed was himself. As a young man, losing his voice for an extended period threatened his livelihood as a salesman. Because nothing helped, Cayce consulted a hypnotist. Under hypnosis, his voice returned, and he was able to prescribe a treatment that resolved his disorder. As the word spread about his "gift" for diagnosing illnesses and prescribing treatments, more doctors requested his help. Although initially reluctant to do so, Cayce ultimately provided more than 14,000 psychic readings during his lifetime, more than 9,000 of which concerned medical subjects. Most of his readings, representing upwards of 900,000 pages of material, were transcribed and are currently available to the public.

In a typical reading, Cayce would induce his own trance and then answer questions directed to him about the patient's medical conditions. His diagnoses did not rely upon any information about the patient provided in advance. The patient's physical presence was not even needed. Cayce needed only the patient's address or location at the time of the reading. While in his trance, Cayce could comment on the weather and other aspects of the patient's physical surroundings. Cayce was never evaluated by scientists under controlled conditions. He became reluctant to have his abilities tested after skeptics—in the name of science—stuck pins in him, pierced his cheek with a hat pin, and pried off a fingernail to see if he was faking his trance.

Cayce recommended diverse therapies that were always safe. They did not belong exclusively to any specific medical tradition (e.g., allopathic medicine, osteopathy, homeopathy, etc.) and could be obscure past remedies or entirely new therapeutic approaches. As such, it was often difficult for patients to find a given health-care professional able to implement the full gamut of Cayce's therapeutic armamentarium. To address this need, a hospital in Virginia Beach, Virginia, was built with the support of investors who had benefited financially from Cayce's readings. However, because these investors did not heed Cayce's warnings about the pending 1929 stock market crash, the hospital was soon forced to close. Nearly 60 years after Cayce's 1945 death, his legacy lives on through many sources, including the Edgar Cayce Foundation, the Association of Research and Enlightenment (ARE), and the Cayce-inspired Atlantic University, all of Virginia Beach; the ARE Clinic, located in Phoenix; and the hundreds of books and articles that have been written about him and his readings.

Causes of Disease

Cayce consistently emphasized certain common denominators that promoted, aggravated, or predisposed people to ailments (see accompanying box). Because he emphasized the relationship between these factors, a mind–body–spirit perspective, and maintaining a preventive focus, Cayce has been called the father of modern holistic medicine.

Spinal Cord Dysfunction

Cayce provided scores of readings for people with spinal cord dysfunction, especially multiple sclerosis (MS) (14) and to a lesser degree SCI (15). To understand better his SCI approaches, it is necessary to review his MS approaches also. Cayce offered no quick cures for spinal cord dysfunction. His therapies required patience, perseverance, and determination.

Cayce believed that the key therapeutic, nervous-system-nurturing factor needed for many neurological disorders was gold, an element that often was inadequately assimilated from the diet. Cayce's primary MS therapy involved administering gold's vibrational energy though one of two mild electrotherapy devices discussed below. He also encouraged meditation or other contemplative practices during the electrotherapy sessions. Finally,

Edgar Cayce's Disease Common Denominators

According to Cayce, diseases often had certain causal common denominators:

- *Poor assimilation:* Occurs when the nutrients and energies required for building new cells and tissues are not supplied, adequately absorbed, or efficiently used.

- *Poor elimination:* Whether through the intestinal tract, bladder and kidneys, skin pores, or lungs, results in the buildup of toxic substances.

- *Poor diet:* Especially lacking fresh fruits and vegetables, compromises health.

- *Improper acid-alkaline balance:* Adversely affects electrochemical communication between cells, including nerve impulses.

- *Spinal dislocations and lesions:* Affect nerve impulses that could directly or indirectly affect every part of the body.

- *Nervous system imbalance:* Adversely affects the entire body. A healthy nervous system requires the assimilation of key nutrients and hormones secreted from glands.

- *Circulatory system imbalance:* Adversely affects the supply of nutrients through the body and the removal of waste products.

- *Glandular malfunction:* Affects the secretion of key hormones required for cellular functions, including the absorption of key nutrients and minerals.

- *Stress and overexertion:* Aggravates physical and mental disorders.

- *Infection:* Especially in combination with other factors.

- *Attitudes, emotions, and karma:* Cayce believed in mind–body–spirit healing, in which your mental attitudes and emotions affect your physical health. In addition, he believed in the role of past-life karmic influences in health, especially in physical disability.

Cayce recommended that patients be massaged after the sessions, using combinations of specific oils and with circular motions starting at the base of the skull, working down both sides of the spine to the legs and feet, and finishing with the arms and hands.

Although it seemed fairly radical at the time, Cayce also suggested what now essentially is considered today's healthy diet, emphasizing low fat, reduced sugar intake, roughage, fresh fruits and vegetables, whole grains, seafood and poultry, and no fried foods. He stressed B vitamins in treating neurological problems and encouraged iodine supplementation, believing that the mineral affected all endocrine glands, not just the thyroid. In an attempt to assess Cayce's recommendations in contemporary times, the Meridian Institute in Virginia Beach carried out a small pilot study (16), which suggested that people who followed Cayce's MS-healing protocol over a six-month period had improved health and reduced symptomatology.

Compared to MS, Cayce provided readings for relatively few people with SCI, because most individuals with serious injuries did not live long in his lifetime—at least not until infection-fighting antibiotics began to become available near the end of his life. In general, Cayce's SCI recommendations were similar to his MS therapies. Designed to promote neuronal health, they included electrotherapy devices to introduce the vibrational energy of gold or other substances into the body, gentle massage using specific oil combinations, and his healthy diet. In addition, Cayce suggested that gentle manipulations from an osteopath specializing in nerve disorders could relieve pressures and promote functioning. Again, no quick cures were offered; improvements would require long-term persistence and patience.

Electrotherapy Devices

Cayce believed that the body was an intricate electromagnetic energy system that must be kept in balance to maintain health. Treatments that help one regain the right balance would facilitate the body's inherent healing potential. To help patients regain balance, Cayce often recommended using the "wet cell battery" and "radial appliance." (17) These devices were constructed based on information in his readings, and each was recommended in nearly a thousand readings for a wide variety of disorders, including spinal cord dysfunction.

Basically, the *wet cell battery*, composed of nickel and copper poles suspended in an electrolytic solution, produces a very low, direct current. Although electrode placement varied depending on the patient, the negative nickel electrode often was attached just above and to the right of the navel, and the positive copper electrode to one of four spinal locations (specifically, in the C1-2, T1-2, T-9, or L-4 regions).

Although it looks like a battery, the *radial appliance* produces no electrical charge of its own. Cayce said it acts like a magnet that draws energy from one part of the body and redistributes to other areas. The appliance's capacitor-like design consists of two steel rods separated by glass and surrounded by carbon. After the core is chilled in ice water, the appliance becomes "electronized" and then can affect the body's electromagnetic energy system. Although electrode placement varied, the appliance's flow of energy was often routed through an electrode to the navel area as above and returned through one attached to a wrist or ankle. For both appliances, if the patient needed gold's vibrational energy, the energy flow was routed through a jar containing a solution of gold chloride. The gold's vibration was then picked up and routed to the body.

Homeopathic Gold Alternative

Rather than to go through the effort with Cayce's vibrational technique, it has been suggested that some individuals may benefit simply from acquiring gold vibrational energy through taking the homeopathic remedy Aurum met (or metallium; a Google search will turn up many citations for this homeopathic agent).

Conclusions

Given how many of Cayce's insights have been uncannily perceptive for myriad disorders, a closer examination of his therapeutic approaches for spinal cord dysfunction seems warranted.

Additional Readings and Resources

Books

Delany D. *The Edgar Cayce Way of Overcoming Multiple Sclerosis: Vibratory Medicine.* Hampton, VA: Meridian Publications, 1999.

Karp RA. *The Edgar Cayce Encyclopedia of Healing*. New York: Warner Books, 1999.
McMillin D, Richards DG. *The Radial Appliance & Wet Cell Battery—Two Electro-therapeutic Devices Recommended by Edgar Cayce*. Virginia Beach, VA: Lifeline Press, 1995.
Sugrue T. *There Is a River—The Story of Edgar Cayce*. New York: Henry Holt, 1942.
Stern J. *Edgar Cayce—The Sleeping Prophet*. Virginia Beach, VA: ARE Press, 1999.
Reilly HJ, Brod RH. *The Edgar Cayce Handbook for Health through Drugless Therapy*. Virginia Beach, VA: ARE Press, 1996.

Internet

Meridian Institute for Researching Edgar Cayce's Holistic Philosophies: www.meridianinstitute.com
Baar Products: Official Supplier of Edgar Cayce Products: www.baar.com

REFERENCES

1. Bellavite P, Signorini A. *Homeopathy: A Frontier in Medical Science*. Berkeley, Calif., North Atlantic Books, 1995.
2. Chapman EH, Weintraub RJ, Milburn MA, et al. Homeopathic treatment of mild traumatic brain injury: A randomized, double-blind, placebo-controlled clinical trial. *J Head Trauma Rehabil* 1999; 14: 521–542.
3. An Oklahoma HMO goes herbal. *Natural Health* January–February, 1999, 23.
4. McIntyre M. Alternative licensing for herbal medicine-like products in the European Union. *J Altern Complement Med* 1999; 5: 110–113.
5. Lazarou J, Pomeranz BH, Corey PN, Incidence of adverse drug reactions in hospitalized patients: a meta-analysis of prospective studies. *JAMA* 1998; 279: 1200–1205.
6. Johnston L. Human spinal cord injury: new and emerging approaches to treatment. *Spinal Cord* 2001; 39: 609–613.
7. Edwards V. Aromatherapy for quadriplegics: a case study. *Aromatic Thymes* Spring 1999; 7.
8. Bach E. Heal Thyself, in The Bach Flower Remedies. The Unique Healing Treatment: Why it Works and How to Benefit from Its 38 Powerful Essences. New Canaan, Conn.: Keats Publishing, 1997.
9. Wright MS. *Flower Essences: Reordering Our Understanding and Approach to Illness and Health*. Warrenton, Va.: Perelandra, 1988.
10. Cram J. Effects of Two Flower Essences on High Intensity Environmental Stimulation and EMF. *Proceedings International Society for the Study of Subtle Energies & Energy Medicine* 2000; 31–33.
11. Cram J. Flower Essence Therapy in the Treatment of Major Depression: Preliminary Findings. *Townsend Letter* 2001; 213: 109–110.
12. Wright MS. *The Human Electrical System and Flower Essences* [videotape]. Warrenton, Va.: Perelandra, 1996.
13. Gurudas. *Flower Essences and Vibrational Healing*. San Rafael, Calif: Cassandra Press, 1989.

14. *Multiple Sclerosis Volumes 1–7*. Circulating Files: Extracts from the Edgar Cayce Readings. Association for Research and Enlightenment (www.are. cayce.com).

15. *Paralysis: Spine Injury Volumes. 1–2*. Circulating Files: Extracts from the Edgar Cayce Readings. Association for Research and Enlightenment (www.are. cayce.com).

16. Meridian Institute. Multiple sclerosis: A report on a Research/Treatment Program Based on the Edgar Cayce readings (www.meridianinstitute.com/ msreport.htm).

17. McMillin D, Richards DG. *The Radial Appliance and Wet Cell Battery—Two Electrotherapeutic Devices Recommended by Edgar Cayce*. Virginia Beach, Va.: Lifeline Press, 1995.

5

Bodywork

CHIROPRACTIC HEALING

Get knowledge of the spine, for this is the requisite for many diseases.
—Hippocrates, the Father of Medicine

A number of years ago, I helped the then PVA president over a curb in the wheelchair-challenging French Quarter of New Orleans. It didn't matter that I routinely worked out at the gym or had aided many wheelchair-using colleagues in the past; this time, I hurt my back. Because of the often awkward nature of such assistance, many caregivers and friends of wheelchair users have had similar experiences.

Overall, back pain is a huge societal problem. For example, 85% of us will be disabled by it sometime, and at any point in time, 7% of adults are suffering from a bout of back pain lasting more than two weeks. It is the second most frequent reason people use the health-care system and the most common cause of work loss and disability. Experts have endorsed chiropractic as one of the most effective ways of treating such pain, discouraging traditional approaches of bed rest, medication, and surgery as counterproductive. Most notably, a 1997 U.S. Agency for Health Care Policy (AHCP) report stated, "Chiropractic is now recognized as the principal source of one of the few treatments recommended by national evidence-based guidelines for the treatment of low-back pain, spinal manipulation" (1, p. 119).

With 35 million Americans visiting 60,000 chiropractors each year, chiropractic is the nation's third-largest health-care profession after medicine and dentistry. Of these people, 70% use chiropractic for back pain; 25% for head, neck, and extremity pain; and 5% for other disorders. Because of its popularity, including among individuals with physical disabilities, chiropractic should no longer be considered alternative medicine but rather a key component of our healthcare system that synergistically complements, not opposes, conventional medicine.

Chiropractic can help caregivers who put their backs in harm's way, and as discussed below can also enhance the wellness of some people with spinal cord injury (SCI) and other disabilities, whose wheelchair living (e.g., transfers, bad posture, imbalanced muscle development, etc.) aggravates physical problems that are amenable to chiropractic treatment.

Definition

Chiropractic focuses on diagnosing and treating musculoskeletal disorders that affect the nervous system, and as a consequence, general health. More specifically, the Association of Chiropractic Colleges defines chiropractic as

> A healthcare discipline that emphasizes the inherent recuperative power of the body to heal itself *without the use of drugs or surgery* (italics added). The practice of chiropractic focuses on the relationship between structure (primarily spine) and function (as coordinated by the nervous system) and how that relationship affects the preservation and restoration of health. In addition, doctors of chiropractic recognize the value and responsibility of working in cooperation with other healthcare practitioners when in the best interest of the patients. (2, p. 57)

Chiropractic's core philosophy differs from conventional medicine, which believes we are the sum of our body parts (e.g., organs, cells, or molecules) and that if we fix the parts, the body will be repaired. In contrast, chiropractic grew out of a holistic *vitalism* philosophy, which says that the body has an innate life force (e.g., like qi or prana in Eastern healing traditions) that flows down from the brain with the nervous system and out from the spine to the periphery. Like fixing a garden-hose kink, chiropractic adjusts musculoskeletal distortions that inhibit this flow, and by so doing enhances wellness.

History

Chiropractic procedures have been a part of humankind's healing armamentarium since time immemorial, including use by ancient

Chinese, Egyptian, and Greek civilizations. Both Hippocrates (460–
377 B.C.) and the influential Roman physician Galen (A.D. 129–199)
recommended vertebral adjustments to relieve ailments.

The founder of modern chiropractic was Daniel David Palmer
(Figure 5-1A) (1845–1913), a self-educated man in medicine and
science who practiced in Davenport, Iowa. In 1895, through vertebral manipulation, he restored the hearing of his building's janitor,
who had been deaf since a back accident 17 years earlier. This
incident gave birth to chiropractic, the term coined from the Greek
words *praxis* and *cheir*, meaning treatment by hand.

Much of the credit for chiropractic's growth was due to the
organizational leadership of Palmer's son, Bartlett Joshua Palmer
(Figure 5-1B) (1881–1961), who at age 21 took over and built up
the now well-known Palmer School of Chiropractic in Davenport.
He was an innovator, who, for example, integrated nascent x-ray
technology into the profession, and was an effective chiropractic
promoter and defender. He cultivated and lobbied national figures

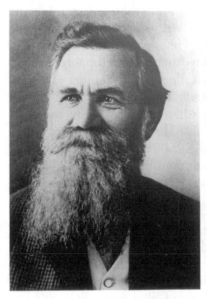 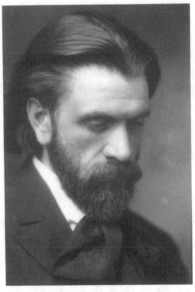

A   B

Figure 5-1   The founder of today's chiropractic Daniel David Palmer **(A)** and
son Bartlett Joshua Palmer, who developed discipline **(B)**. (Photo provided by
Palmer College of Chiropractic Archives, Davenport, IA.)

and U.S. presidents, and even employed future President Ronald Reagan as a broadcaster at his World of Chiropractic (WOC) radio station. Gradually, states approved chiropractic; Minnesota was the first (1905), and Louisiana the last (1974).

Chiropractic faced vociferous opposition from organized medicine. Because the allopathic medicine discipline did not include a spinal-manipulation focus—preferring its pharmaceutical and surgical approaches—it minimized the benefits that could accrue from this focus emphasized by a competing discipline. In defense of organized medicine—which had made huge health-care advances as it transitioned into the 20th century and cleaned up its own house by imposing rigorous professional standards—many of the early chiropractic profession's actions, infighting, and lax standards fueled criticism. Chiropractic emergence was also handicapped, however, because it did not advocate drugs, and therefore could not cultivate strong financial, pharmaceutical-industry allies. Organized medicine was forced to back down when a landmark 1987 federal antitrust ruling found the American Medical Association (AMA) guilty of a prolonged and systematic attempt to undermine completely the chiropractic profession, often using highly dishonest methods. By stopping the major source of organized resistance, this case ushered in a new era of cooperation between physicians and chiropractors. In recent decades, federal actions have increasingly supported chiropractic, including the 1974 authorization to the Council of Chiropractic Education to accredit schools; the aforementioned AHCP endorsement of chiropractic to treat lower back pain; the 1996 decision by the National Institutes of Health to fund chiropractic research; and President Bill Clinton's 2000 mandate that chiropractic be made available to all active-duty military personnel.

Education

Facilitating its current acceptance, the chiropractic profession has adopted strict educational standards, comparable in rigor but different in focus from medical education. Although the basic-science components of both professions are equivalent in study time, chiropractic emphasizes musculoskeletal and neuroanatomical systems over medicine's pharmacological and surgical priorities. Furthermore, in contrast to medicine's broad clinical preparation, chiropractic clinical training is specialized, focusing on the profession's unique diagnostic and treatment methods, which can only be mastered through extensive, hands-on practice.

Procedures

Chiropractors focus on correcting disordered vertebral joints, which include vertebrae and their bony projections (called facet joints and spinous or transverse processes), shock-absorbing cartilage discs, muscles, ligaments, and nervous tissue. *Subluxations*—abnormalities of this vertebral complex—affect health by impinging on nerve roots as they exit the complex through channels called intervertebral foramen. Because of the complex's inherent intricacy, subluxations can result from numerous, interacting factors that upset the complex's homeostatic equilibrium, for instance, from unbalanced muscle tension that pulls a vertebra out of alignment with its neighbors. In turn, a specific subluxation can create a chain reaction, affecting other parts of the spinal column. For example, neck pain may be the secondary consequence of a pelvic misalignment.

Chiropractic emphasizes noninvasive therapies, such as manual treatments, physical therapy, exercise programs, nutritional advice, orthotics, and lifestyle modification. The most common procedure is the spinal adjustment, accomplished through diverse techniques. For example, with spinal *manipulation*, using the vertebral projections as levers, a carefully measured force is rapidly applied to the joint that carries it past its voluntary range of motion but still well within the range permitted by nature. The commonly heard "crack" is actually a vacuum-created nitrogen bubble bursting within the joint. In contrast, with spinal *mobilization* procedures, the joint remains within its passive range of movement. Depending on the problem's acute or chronic nature, multiple treatment sessions often are needed, 6 to 10 being the average.

Studies show that the chiropractic risks are minimal. For example, a 1996 RAND Corporation study concluded that 1.5 serious complications occur from every million cervical manipulations. By comparison, there are 1,000 serious complications per million from taking over-the-counter painkillers.

Chiropractic and SCI

People with disabilities frequently use chiropractic. For example, a pilot study by the Kessler Institute in New Jersey indicated 23% of people with SCI with chronic pain had used chiropractic (3).

Dr. Julet Hutchens (Figure 5-2), a chiropractor who practices with medical doctors and physical therapists, discusses potential SCI benefits:

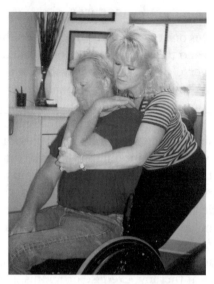

Figure 5-2   Dr. Julet Hutchens, a chiropractor in Colorado, adjusts her husband Eddy to aid in his range of movement. (Photo taken by Laurance Johnston.)

I have treated patients with spinal cord injury and dysfunction for four years, the first of which was my husband Eddy, a wheelchair athlete and an associate member of Mountain States chapter of the Paralyzed Veterans of America. When I met him, he had been paralyzed 16 years due to an automobile accident, in which he sustained a complete T-10 spinal-cord transection.

I adjust Eddy usually 1 to 2 times per month depending on his activity and discomfort level. I keep the majority of my adjustments to him and other paralyzed patients above the injury level. However, occasionally, I will perform more passive types of mobilization to the pelvis, low back, and lower extremities. Eddy says the adjustments give him instant relief to shoulder problems, upper/mid-back and rib pain, and neck pain. A Denver Rolling Nuggets basketball player, he recommends chiropractic treatments to his teammates to ensure their continued full range of movement above and below the injury site.

I often treat shoulder and rib-related injuries in individuals with paralysis that result from their excessive shoulder and arm use associated with frequent wheelchair transfers. Often, a repetitive-use injury occurs, which, if not taken care of, can lead to more severe shoulder problems, even requiring surgery. Chiropractic treats the shoulders and ribs, giving the patient relief. And with any repetitive-use injury, strengthening exercises reinforce adjustments, preventing future injuries.

As with any person sitting for long time periods, posture becomes an issue in wheelchair users. Most end up with neck and upper-back pain due to bad posture. When we sit for a long time, we tend to slump forward, placing extra stress on the neck and upper back. When I observe wheelchair athletes, I see them leaning forward, resting their arms on their legs, or leaning slightly forward and to the side, resting on a wheel. Such posture places extra stress on the neck and upper back, and, as a result, the muscles around the spine become weak and those in the chest become tighter. These changes cause an imbalance between front and back muscles, which can lead to pain. I work with the patient to rebuild muscle balance, and restore motion in the spine that is restricted from such imbalance. Teaching patients the difference between good and bad posture is especially important so that they become aware of the small changes they can make to alleviate some of their neck and back issues.

Active individuals with paralysis will develop a strong upper body to compensate for their inability to balance themselves through the use of abdominal, leg, and lower-back muscles as an able-bodied person would. Because of this upper-body reliance, we want to keep it in good working order, which is accomplished through a strong chiropractic and stretching and strengthening programs. Shoulder or neck pain can impair one's ability to not only transfer in or out of a wheelchair but also to push it, limiting overall mobility.

Adjustments, muscle work, and exercises keep the spine, shoulders, ribs, and shoulder blades moving as they should in a painless, full range of motion. These methods keep the joints lubricated, discs between the vertebrae from deteriorating, and muscles and ligaments strong and balanced. At the same time, it loosens muscles. Overall, because they will be healthier, feel better, and have more energy, all wheelchair users should receive regular bodywork.

When I treat patients with SCI, arthritis that causes joint fusing, post-polio, or cerebral palsy, I adapt my treatment to accommodate the patient. Depending on their disability, I treat patients in their wheelchair, or if comfortable, I will help them transfer to a treatment table.

I try to choose the optimal treatment for the specific patient, some of which are more passive or aggressive than others. I also x-ray all patients with SCI to see exactly what is going on in their spine, shoulders, etcetera. With SCI, the body compensates in one area for the lack of motion in another. Because such compensation can be observed through x-rays, the patient can be more effectively treated.

Conclusions

Most healing traditions have something valuable to offer, yet at the same time have limitations in scope. For example, allopathic medicine emphasizes valuable pharmaceutical and surgical interventions, whereas chiropractic focuses on musculoskeletal system mechanisms that medicine has ignored. Chiropractic has much to offer individuals with SCI who are often plagued with overuse injuries.

Additional Readings and Resources

Books

Chapman-Smith DA. *The Chiropractic Profession: Its Education, Practice, Research and Future Directions.* Toronto: Harmony Printing, 2000.

Internet

American Chiropractic Association: www.amerchiro.org

CRANIOSACRAL THERAPY

Craniosacral therapy is a gentle, hands-on bodywork procedure for evaluating and enhancing the functioning of the craniosacral system, a physiological system surrounding the brain and spinal cord. Therapy advocates believe this system influences the whole body by affecting the brain and spinal cord, as well as the brain's pituitary and pineal glands. As such, the craniosacral system serves as a core function in that the entire body's health depends on its well-being. As a core function, the therapy has the ability to treat a wide range of disorders and physical disability, including spinal cord injury.

History

Craniosacral therapy evolved from osteopathic medicine, with its musculoskeletal emphasis. In the early 1900s, osteopathic physician William Sutherland concluded that skull bones are not firmly fixed but can move relative to each other. With these observations, he developed a treatment called cranial osteopathy. In recent years, Dr. John Upledger (Figure 5-3) further developed Sutherland's observations and incorporated them into a treatment now called craniosacral therapy (4). Upledger's interest was whetted early in his career. While assisting a neurosurgeon in the removal of plaque from a patient's spinal cord membrane, Upledger observed the membrane pulsating in spite of his best efforts to keep it still. This was his first observation of the craniosacral rhythm. He later researched this phenomenon for eight years as a professor of biomechanics at Michigan State University. To transfer his research findings more effectively to consumers, in 1985 he established the

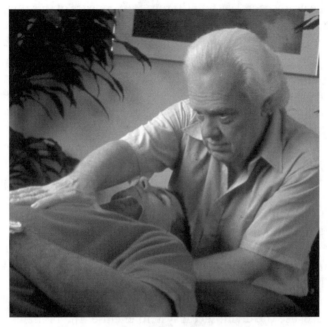

Figure 5-3 Dr. John Upledger, developer of craniosacral therapy, treating patient. (Photo provided by Upledger Institute, Palm Beach Gardens, FL.)

Upledger Institute in Palm Beach Gardens, Florida (5). Since then, many have been trained in craniosacral therapy, including osteopaths, medical doctors, chiropractors, psychologists, dentists, physical therapists, acupuncturists, and massage therapists.

The Craniosacral System

The spinal cord is surrounded by a protective, three-layered membrane system (the meninges) that lies within the vertebral column. The outside layer is called the *dura mater;* the middle layer the *arachnoid membrane;* and the innermost layer the *pia mater.* The inside layer is tightly attached to the spinal cord, whereas cerebrospinal fluid is between the other sections. In addition to providing nutrients, the lubricating cerebrospinal fluid allows the membrane layers to glide in relation to one another as the spine bends and twists. The tough dura mater protects everything inside it, including the brain and spinal cord.

The craniosacral system (Figure 5-4) consists of this membrane system, the enclosed cerebrospinal fluid, the physiological structures that control fluid input and outflow, and related bones. It is a semi-enclosed biological hydraulic system encompassing the brain and spinal cord. Within the system, the cerebrospinal fluid rhythmically pulses at a rate of about ten cycles per minute. This is independent of heart or respiratory rhythms. The craniosacral system's fluid barrier is the dura mater, which also composes the skull's inside lining. Upledger's research indicates that the skull bones must be slightly moving continuously to accommodate the fluid pressure changes within this semi-closed hydraulic system. The membrane barrier is also attached to the upper neck vertebrae, the lower back sacrum, the tailbone, and the openings in the spinal column where nerves go out to the body. Any occurrence that interferes with the membrane's ability to accommodate the rhythmically fluctuating fluid pressures and volumes is a potential problem.

The object of craniosacral therapy is to find areas of restricted movement that compromise function and reestablish normal movement. Because the craniosacral system encloses the brain and spinal

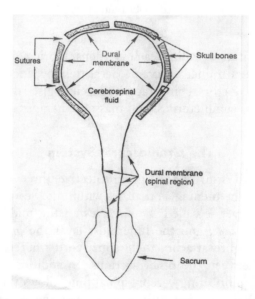

Figure 5-4   Key features of craniosacral system. (Illustration from Upledger JE. *Your Inner Physician and You: Craniosacral Therapy & Somatoemotional Release.* Berkeley, CA: North Atlantic Books, 1997. Used with permission.)

cord, it influences the entire nervous system, affecting many body functions. These include the brain's important pituitary and pineal glands, which in turn have the potential to affect the body's entire hormonal balance.

Skull-Bone Movement?

Mainstream medicine has criticized craniosacral therapy under the assumption that skull bones permanently fuse during infancy. However, this dogma is not universally accepted by medicine. For example, in parts of Europe, it is taught that the skull bones do, indeed, have movement potential. Upledger feels that the axiom about fused skull bones may have come from the routine practice of using long-dead cadavers treated with preservative chemicals for anatomical examinations. He says that fresh, unpreserved sutures (the skull bone edges) are full of dynamic tissue, nerves, and blood vessels, consistent with a flexible system allowing some movement. In contrast, the sutures from old preserved skulls appear calcified. Upledger says most neurosurgeons have not observed the craniosacral rhythm because most surgery penetrates the membrane barrier required to maintain the rhythm.

Hands-On Process

During craniosacral therapy, trained therapists use a light touch equivalent to a nickel's weight, and feel the rhythmic motion of the cerebrospinal fluid within the craniosacral system. Therapists check the rate, amplitude, symmetry, and quality of this wavelike motion in places where the craniosacral membrane barrier attaches to bones such as the skull, sacrum, and tailbone. Any restrictions or blockages are treated with light-touch adjustments. A restriction in one part of the craniosacral system can affect the entire system, so treatment may involve working at a point distant from the overt symptom. By assisting the hydraulic forces in the craniosacral system and in turn improving central nervous system (CNS) functioning, treatment facilitates the body's innate, self-healing mechanisms.

Spinal Cord Injury

Most of the many individuals with SCI who have been treated by the Upledger Institute have reported some improvement, ranging from modest to fairly dramatic. Change takes place with motor function, bowel and bladder control, spasticity management, and overall well-being and ease. Because patients are usually several years postinjury, improvement is not attributed to residual, ongoing functional improvement often observed in the first year after injury.

As in the case of many health-care professionals using substantial hands-on bodywork, experienced craniosacral therapists feel as if they can "read" the body. For example, they can localize the level of injury without other information. Furthermore, they often note the presence of secondary and tertiary injury sites resulting from the mechanics and vector forces of impact. A C-4 quadriplegic, for example, may have experienced secondary trauma at the T-5 level.

Upledger says initial trauma results in edema, in which a burst of cerebrospinal fluid results in tissue separation that heals with fibrous scarring. "It is like a copper wire after being hit with a hammer; it won't conduct as well" (personal communication, August 1998). Because this secondary damage occurs relatively soon after injury, Upledger believes that to get fluids moving, patients should receive treatment soon after injury.

Jackie's Story

Jackie became an incomplete quadriplegic after a car accident. He has been treated several times at the Upledger facility and emphatically states that "they have helped me more than anyone ever has before. I now have much more feeling and muscle control." Jackie now walks without the full leg brace that was previously needed. He is a man that likes to "work hard and play hard," and his improved trunk muscles, which are critical for balance, allow him to use a three-wheel motorcycle once again. He distinctly remembers the moment on the therapy table that he first regained some feeling in his left hip. "The tingle felt like the sensation when you try to move a leg that has gone to sleep."

Conclusions

A gentle hands-on bodywork therapy, craniosacral therapy has considerable potential for restoring or enhancing some quality-of-life function in individuals with spinal cord injury.

Additional Readings and Resources

Books

Upledger JE. *Your Inner Physician and You: Craniosacral Therapy and Somatoemotional Release*. Berkeley, Calif.: North Atlantic Books, 1997.

Internet

The Upledger Institute's Craniosacral Therapy Program: www.upledger.com

CHRONOLOGICALLY CONTROLLED DEVELOPMENTAL THERAPY

Chronologically controlled developmental therapy (CCDT) consists of a combination of fairly standard physical therapy techniques. Its uniqueness relates to how these techniques are applied, their sequence, and the patient's passive involvement. This treatment was developed by Ed Snapp, a highly credentialed physical therapist who acquired polio when he was 18. Snapp has visionary, paradigm-expanding perspectives on how the central nervous system functions after injury, and a Zenlike appreciation of the body, in which he obtains an array of valuable diagnostic information by assessing subtle aspects of movement and reactions to stimulus.

Treatment

CCDT targets a wide range of neurological disorders, including spinal cord injury (SCI), postpolio syndrome, head injury, cerebral palsy and various developmental disorders. Basically, CCDT consists of various physical therapies performed in a specific, defined sequence, including pressure stimulation, hydrotherapy, light-touch massage, and movements on an oil table. Unlike many rehabilitation programs, the therapies are passive—the therapy is done to you; you exert no effort. You are encouraged to let go of any conscious effort to control the situation. To keep your nervous system from being distracted from nontherapy stimulation, the procedures occur in a environment that minimizes distraction (e.g., under dim light, no talking, etc.).

Spinal Cord Injury

Many with SCI have been treated with CCDT, and if they persist with the treatment, often significant functional recovery has accrued over time. For example, Nick fell 25 feet from a hunting platform and crushed his spine in the thoracic/lumbar region. Although two years later his legs were jammed with extreme spasms, after several years of treatment, Nick was walking with crutches and short braces.

Snapp notes that CCDT gradually restores function in the next lower spinal segment.

> Patients with T-5-12 injuries seem to be the most responsive, even with long-standing paralysis. Most frequently, the primary response is the return of the spinal extensors (back muscles used for sitting erect) on both sides of the spinal column. The next expected functions are respectively (a) the ability to intensify the unilateral contraction of the spinal muscles when turning the head or moving the head from side to side; (b) the adductor muscles (legs together) of the hips from an abducted position (legs apart); and (c) the beginning of hip flexion and adduction from a position of moderate abduction and outward hip rotation. (6)

Theory

Although procedures are relatively straightforward, CCDT theory is not. Basically, CCDT focuses on activating intact, but dormant, neurons and pathways. Scientists now believe that most nonpenetrative injuries (i.e., injuries other than from gunshots or stabbing) that have been clinically classified as complete are neuronally incomplete injuries. In other words, often intact but dormant neurons exist across the injury site. Animal studies suggest that only a small percentage of functioning neurons are needed to have substantial physical function. As such, if we can activate some dormant, intact neurons, considerable function potentially could be regained.

CCDT is based on a thought-provoking theory involving concepts of evolutionary development. Basically, turning on dormant neurons requires a sequence of cues that mimic events from our early fetal and infant development. In turn, these developmental cues reflect a genetic memory of our evolutionary development. If a fully developed neuron has been turned off, its reactivation requires that it receive and sense external cues in a defined sequence correlated to the neuron's initial development. There is no avenue to deliver these cues except through the peripheral senses—the basis of CCDT's physical therapy program. Out-of-sequence cues will not work, which is why Snapp believes so many more traditional rehabilitation programs have limited outcomes. It is like pulling a computer plug. The computer's circuits remain intact, but the program is lost. To be reinstalled, the computer must be rebooted, which involves a sequential series of steps. Likewise, neurological dysfunctions often result from a deprogramming of specific portions of the central nervous system. In the same fashion that a disk can be used to reboot a computer, an appropriate external cue will trigger information residing within a nervous system's genetic code. This information will then be reprogrammed back into the operating system in the same order it was learned in the embryonic nervous system.

CCDT clinics are located in Columbus, Mississippi, and Spokane, Washington.

Conclusions

Chronologically controlled developmental therapy, consisting of commonly used physical therapies carried out in a defined sequence, provides function-restoring benefits for various neurological disorders, including spinal cord injury.

Additional Readings and Resources

Internet

Chronologically Controlled Development Therapy: www.futuresunlimited.com

REFERENCES

1. Cherkin DC, Mootz RD. *Chiropractic in the United States: Training, Practice, and Research*. AHCPR Publication No. 98-N002. Rockville, MD, December 1997.
2. Chapman-Smith DA. *The Chiropractic Profession: Its Education, Practice, Research and Future Directions*. Toronto: Harmony Printing, 2000.
3. Nayak S, Matheis RJ, Agostinelli MA, et al. The use of complementary and alternative therapies for chronic pain following spinal cord injury: a pilot study. *J Spinal Cord Med* 2001; 24(1): 54–62.

4. Upledger JE. *Your Inner Physician and You: Craniosacral Therapy and Somatoemotional Release*. Berkeley, Calif.: North Atlantic Books, 1997.
5 The Upledger Institute's Craniosacral Therapy Program (www.upledger.com).
6. Chronologically Controlled Development Therapy (www.futuresunlimited.com)

6

Dolphin-Assisted Therapy

IS THERE A DOLPHIN IN THE HOUSE?

In alternative-medicine circles, dolphins have been cited as having special capabilities that enhance healing potential in people with a physical disability, including spinal cord injury (SCI). Throughout the ages, man has had a special fascination with dolphins. This relationship continues to be acknowledged today by many diverse sources. Dr. John Lilly determined in his studies of the human brain and interspecies communication the possibility that man may rank behind the dolphin in terms of cerebral development. The U.S. Navy has also recognized the dolphin's intelligence capabilities and has been using them for highly specialized missions for many years. Even ancient cultures speak of connective links to the dolphins. One such culture existing to this day is an Australian aborigine tribe known as the Dolphin People. They believe their ancestors were the souls of dolphins who were slaughtered by sharks and then reborn as the first humans.

The Dolphin

Dolphins are highly social creatures, living in groups of varying size called pods. They are mammals who nurse their young and must surface to breathe. In the wild, dolphins can live up to 50 years. Like humans, dolphins have a large, complex brain, especially the area associated with higher cognitive functioning. Dolphins navigate through their aqueous environment using a highly sophisticated sonar system. They emit a focused blast of ultrasound vibrations, which reflect off objects before returning to them. Their powerful sonar can penetrate up to three feet through sand and mud with resolution significant enough to distinguish between a dime and a penny. Due to this power, scientists believe that dolphins can view the inside of our bodies, similar to sonograms performed on pregnant women. Indeed, dolphins are fascinated with pregnant women, homing in on the unborn fetus. Furthermore, they often focus on individuals' specific areas of impairment, as well as on places containing tumors. Often people who swim with the dolphins can feel themselves being scanned. As if bypassing the ears, the sound resonates in the bones, traveling up the spine.

Dolphin-Assisted Therapy

Dolphins appear to facilitate healing through mechanisms not readily reconciled with modern medical precepts. People frequently report becoming euphoric after swimming with these loving, graceful, joyous creatures. In turn, an uplifted spirit seems to infuse beneficial healing effects into the mind and body. Numerous people who have serious illnesses and depression have reported dramatic, long-term, favorable changes in their emotional state. Scientists now know that these emotional changes (which last much longer than the high experienced from the release of endorphins, the body's natural opiates) can initiate a cascade of health-enhancing hormonal and physiological changes. Children with a variety of developmental disabilities have shown remarkable improvements after dolphin-assisted therapy. Learning, cognitive abilities, concentration, communication, and ability to relate to others all improve.

In addition to possessing a direct therapeutic effect, dolphins appear to enhance other therapies. For example, the Upledger Institute in Palm Beach Gardens, Florida, treats individuals with a variety of disorders with dolphin-assisted craniosacral therapy (discussed in the previous chapter of this book). The therapy was completed in the water with, and in near proximity to, the dolphins. Many beneficial effects were observed beyond levels normally realized, including pain reduction, increased ease in breathing, muscle relaxation, enhanced strength and flexibility, increased appetite, and better sleep. Furthermore, the dolphin's sonar echolocation apparently reduced various tissue restrictions, including adhesions resulting from past surgeries, scarring, or trauma.

Spinal Cord Injury

John (Figure 6-1), a paraplegic since 1988, is an actor, writer, poet, and playwright who once worked with Tennessee Williams. He recorded his experiences with dolphin-assisted craniosacral therapy in a journal, including the following:

> Dolphin Therapy this morning, my Lord, what a morning! First we went for a "structured swim" with two pregnant dolphins. The regular stuff, dorsal pulls, imitative games, kisses, and pets. Then into a pool with a dolphin named Tina, a young female, and a very strong girl. Tina would go to my feet and blast energy up from there; it was completely powerful. Suddenly my feet came alive with a pulsing energy. That pulsing energy went through my body and into my lower spinal cord. Every time Tina would blast from my feet, I would get a "therapeutic earthquake" from my first lumbar vertebrae down into my sacrum. All my tissues in the lower part of my body were literally shaking with energy. Talk about sending a shiver up the spine, this was the ultimate.
>
> Next Day: Starting at my feet, there is a constant flow and movement of impulse, an indescribable gyration of synergy that rotates and pulsates, ebbs and flows, buzzes and beats, vibrates and

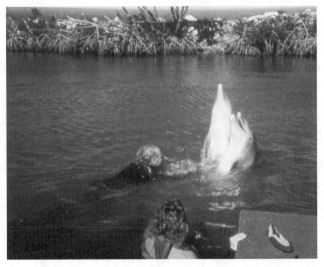

Figure 6-1 John, an individual with SCI, swimming with the dolphins. (Photo provided by Upledger Institute, Palm Beach Gardens, FL.)

harmonizes with a myriad of sensations that move up and down my legs. This is more than I've felt down there since the night I fell out of that tree. And the location is different too . . . this morning, the energy web has moved all the way down into my feet and pulsating upward from there. It is warm, I would say an almost glowing awareness of my feet and legs, tissues and bone. It feels so fine.

How Dolphins Heal

Although no one really knows how and to what degree dolphins heal, a number of both scientific and intuitive speculations have been put forth.

Sound and Vibration

Scientists believe that the dolphin's ultrasound emissions have considerable healing potential from an energy and informational perspective (Figure 6-2). Clinically, ultrasound has been used to promote healing, for diagnostic imaging, and to destroy cataracts and kidney and gallstones. Throughout history, sound—such as music, drumming and chanting—has been used to promote health. Physiologically, we now know that these sounds can influence heart rate, breathing, muscle contractions, memory, and immune function. In terms of energy, the dolphin's ultrasound blast is four times stronger than ultrasound that is used therapeutically in hospitals. Furthermore, the blast is delivered through water, which is 60 times more efficient than air for sound transference, to a body that is three-quarters fluid. It is believed that ultrasound resonance within the cerebrospinal fluid is especially important due to the fluid's key influence on the brain and spinal cord.

Brain Waves

David Cole of Aquathought Foundation has shown that human brain waves shift from high-frequency beta to low-frequency theta waves after a dolphin encounter (1). Beta waves are associated with increased concentration, alertness and enhanced memory function. In contrast, theta waves are associated with enhanced creativity, sensory integration, and altered states of consciousness. For the sake of reference, people exhibit theta waves in the fleeting moments when they drift from consciousness into sleep.

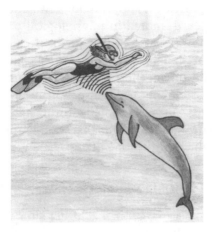

Figure 6-2 Some scientists speculate that the dolphin's therapeutic energy is mediated through human energy fields. (Drawing by Shiara Lightfoot.)

Scientists believe that a brain-wave shift of this nature strengthens the human immune system. Furthermore, research after a dolphin encounter has shown a synchronization of brain-wave activity between the logical, analytical left brain and the intuitive, imaginative right brain. These brain-wave alterations may explain why people view swimming with the dolphins as a transcendental experience. Cole speculates that these brain-wave alterations are facilitated by sonar-induced cavitation (1). Basically, the dolphin's intense sound waves create alternating regions of compression and expansion that form small cell-membrane bubbles. In turn, these bubbles facilitate the transport of key neurological molecules from outside to inside neurons.

Human Energy Fields

Some scientists speculate that the dolphins' therapeutic energy is mediated through human energy fields. According to human-energy-field theory (see chapter 9, Part 2: How Spirituality Can Promote Physical Healing), disease has its origins in the energy field at an atomic level, which then progressively manifests in the molecular, cellular, and body-system levels (2). Conversely, if the energy field is repaired, healing will progress to the physical body. The human energy field responds to stimulus, such as sound, even when the person experiences no conscious awareness of the stimulus and before changes are noted in physiological parameters such as brain waves, blood pressure, and so forth. Because it is theorized that the effects of spinal cord injury are stored in these energy fields, mending the human energy field first will promote the body's healing. Perhaps, dolphins can sense human-energy-field imbalances and adjust their ultrasonic emanations. The dolphin's powerful energy may initiate an appropriate alteration in the human electromagnetic field, which in turn facilitates healing.

Intuitive Perspective

Elan O'Brien, who became a spiritual healer after a transformational experience with dolphins, says these animals' energy represents an alignment with a greater consciousness. According to her, human nervous-system programming usually prevents us from realizing that alignment and expressing the natural order. Dolphins, through their sonar and mudra-like movements, can shift our programming patterns by changing the body's electromagnetic fields. As a result, the body's limited belief structures are opened and changed.

Conclusions

In spite of these speculations, no one truly knows how dolphins mediate healing. Evidence indicates that it is more than a mere psychosomatic, feel-good effect, and most likely represents unknown healing mechanisms beyond traditional medical perspectives. Clearly, evidence suggests it is worthy of further investigation.

Acknowledgment

The assistance of Dr. Russell Bourne is greatly appreciated.

Additional Readings and Resources

Books

Cochrane A, Callen K. *Dolphins and Their Power to Heal*. Rochester, Vt.: Healing Arts Press, 1992.

Internet

Second Annual International Symposium on Dolphin Assisted Therapy, Cancun, Mexico, September 5–8, 1996: www.aquathought.com/idatra

REFERENCES

1. Cole D. Electroencephalographic results of Human-Dolphin Interaction: A Sonophoresis Model. *Second Annual International Symposium on Dolphin Assisted Therapy*, Cancun, Mexico, September 5–8, 1996 (www.aquathought.com/idatra).
2. Hunt V. *Infinite Mind: Science of Human Vibrations of Consciousness*. Malibu, Calif.: Malibu Publishing, 1996.

7

Electromagnetic Healing

MAGNETIC HEALING: OVERVIEW

In the late 18th century, Franz Anton Mesmer used bar magnets and hypnotic "animal magnetism" (hence, mesmerize) to treat patients. Because of the controversy surrounding this procedure, France's King Louis XVI formed a prestigious commission composed of preeminent scientists, including Benjamin Franklin, to investigate Mesmer. This scrutiny ruined Mesmer's career. In an outcome perhaps to be envied by modern scientists whose papers and grants are rejected by their peers, and in a paradoxical twist of fate, commission member Joseph Guillotin's invention later beheaded the king, as well as many other commission members. In contrast, Mesmer died many years later.

Until relatively recently, scientists believed that life was mostly a biochemical process. The idea that magnetic fields could significantly influence living systems seemed far-fetched. Perspectives have shifted rapidly, however, and many scientists now believe that at some level we are fundamentally electromagnetic creatures. This radical paradigm shift has profound medical implications because modern medicine has focused on biochemical processes. If these processes are influenced by our electromagnetic nature, any healing approach that focuses exclusively on them will ultimately be limited.

Life's Magnetic Nature

Examples of life's magnetic nature are now plentiful. Many creatures, such as homing pigeons, butterflies, and bees, navigate using Earth's magnetic field. Even humans can roughly sense magnetic direction. These abilities appear to be mediated in part through a magnetic substance called magnetite, which has been discovered in living tissue, including the human brain. Researchers have found magnetite clusters near the brain's all-important, magnetically sensitive pineal gland, which secretes hormones affecting the entire body. (Interestingly, many people with spinal cord dysfunction—including multiple sclerosis and quadriplegia though not paraplegia—have dysfunctional pineal glands, and as a result lack sensitivity to Earth's profound magnetic influences.)

Not only are we affected by magnetic fields, but we also generate them. For example, we can measure the brain and heart's magnetic fields with instruments called the magnetoencephalograph and magnetocardiogram, respectively. Life's magnetic potential is so great that we can even defy gravity under the right circumstances. For example, scientists can levitate frogs by using high-intensity magnetic fields. When subjected to such strong fields, spinning electrons within the frog align themselves to create cumulatively a small magnetic field. Like a compass needle repulsed by a bar magnet, the large external field repels the frog's small field sufficiently to counteract gravity.

History

Magnetism has always been a part of mankind's healing armamentarium. Many indigenous and ancient civilizations—including the Hebrews, Arabs, Indians, Chinese, Egyptians, and Greeks—used magnets for healing. According to legend, Cleopatra wore a magnetic amulet on her forehead to preserve her youth; this placement put it near the brain's magnetically sensitive pineal gland.

One of the more influential figures in magnetic-healing history was the 15th century physician Paracelsus, who helped to bring medicine out of the Dark Ages. Supposedly, the inspiration for Goethe's Dr. Faustus, who sold his soul to the devil in exchange for knowledge, Paracelsus had visionary insights on the role of energetic forces in healing, including magnetism, and he stated: "Magnetism is the king of all secrets" (1, p. 200). His insights anticipated by nearly 500 years the underlying concepts of modern mind–body disciplines, such as psychoneuroimmunolgy and many holistic approaches. Basically, Paracelsus believed that magnetic force could energize the body and promote self-healing. His work greatly influenced Mesmer.

In America, magnet use soared after the Civil War. People could even order the devices through the Sears & Roebuck catalog.

Turn-of-the-century medical texts devoted chapters to the subject. However, as pharmaceutical approaches revolutionized medicine, magnetic therapy lost its appeal—until recently when the limitations of these approaches became more evident. The magnetic-healing renaissance has been remarkable. Millions of people throughout the world now use magnets, and some cost-conscious health-insurance companies cover the therapy.

How Magnets Work

Magnetism is created primarily by the spin of electrons within a substance. If the spin of sufficient numbers of electrons is aligned, the substance becomes magnetic. Although iron is readily magnetized because of its many surplus electrons, virtually all substances can be magnetized. Natural magnets—lodestones—were created when lava containing iron cooled and was magnetized by Earth's magnetic field. Most magnets now are made by passing a strong surge of direct-current (DC) electricity through an iron bar. Their strength has been greatly increased by combining iron with other elements.

Therapeutic Uses

Magnets are available in a wide range of materials, strengths, and shapes: tiny BB-size ones used by acupuncturists; dime-size; neo-dymium (a rare-earth metal) of extraordinary power; domino; rect-angular block; and flexible magnets of any size and shape. Therapeutic magnets often are cased in ceramic or embedded in an elastic patch or flexible strip. They are incorporated in wrist and back supports, seat and mattress pads, jewelry, and other items, such as shoe inserts and belts.

Many medical applications and scientific studies have used pulsed electromagnetic fields. In these fields, the electric current generating the magnetic field is turned on and off at a specified frequency. Because magnetic fields drop off quickly with distance, the closer the magnet is to the skin the more impact it will have.

Strength

A magnet's therapeutic strength is a function of magnetic flux—measured in gauss—and physical size. For reference, Earth's magnetic field is 0.5 gauss, a refrigerator magnet holding a shopping list about 10 gauss, and a cupboard-door latch magnet about 400.

Therapeutic magnets range from 200 to over 10,000 gauss. Magnet size is also therapeutically important. For example, small neodymium magnets may have strength in excess of 10,000 gauss. However, because their fields can only penetrate a few inches into the body, they are used for treating localized conditions. In contrast, a large block magnet of much lower flux strength may penetrate through the body. Given the importance of size, the profound influence on life of Earth's small 0.5-gauss field is more readily understandable.

Polarity

Although understudied, a magnet's poles appear to exert different healing effects. The north one (the side that attracts the north-pole-seeking end of a compass needle) calms, sedates, and reduces inflammation. In contrast, the south pole stimulates and promotes healing, growth and activity.

How Magnets Affect the Body

Although they are not exactly sure how, scientists believe that magnetic fields perturb the body's own magnetic energy, which in turn triggers more conventional biochemical and physiological mechanisms. Magnetic fields

- Increase blood flow, bringing in more oxygen and nutrients, and flushing away waste products

- Modulate calcium flow through the body, which is essential to many physiological processes. Magnetic fields can attract calcium ions to heal a broken bone or help move calcium away from painful arthritic joints

- Alter the acidity or alkalinity of body fluids, which are often out of balance with illness

- Affect hormone production (including those of the brain's all-important pineal gland), which initiates a cascade of biological effects

- Alter enzyme activity and other biochemical processes, such as the production of ATP, a molecule that provides cellular fuel for the entire body

- Stimulate electromagnetic energy flow through acupuncture meridians

- Alter cell chromosome alignment

Healing Applications

People have used magnetic therapy to treat many ailments. The book *Healing with Magnets* provides an extensive list of these ailments and also of supporting scientific studies (2). General uses include relief of pain and discomfort, reduction of inflammation, improved circulation, the ability to fight infections, reduction of stress, sleep promotion, correction of various central nervous system disorders, overall energy enhancement, acceleration of healing (especially bone fractures), and athletic performance enhancement. Because paralysis aggravates many ailments amenable to magnetic therapy, the therapy may be especially relevant for people with spinal cord injury (SCI) and dysfunction. For example, studies have shown that magnetic therapy is effective in controlling pain, enhancing circulation, promoting wound healing, reducing carpal tunnel syndrome, and other conditions.

Pain

People with spinal cord dysfunction often experience considerable pain for a variety of reasons, including overuse injuries or joint and muscle inactivity. In the long term, painkilling drugs are not the answer. Their effectiveness is limited, the body builds up tolerance, and their side effects hospitalize more than 76,000 people each year. Because of the need, pain has been the most emphasized magnetic-therapy application; numerous studies support its efficacy, including for spinal cord dysfunction (Figure 7-1).

For example, one study focused on the pain associated with postpolio syndrome (3). This study used a double-blind design, the scientific gold-standard for showing effectiveness. The design eliminates the psychological placebo effect because neither physician nor subject knows who receives treatment or who receives placebo control. Physicians strapped either a small, low-intensity magnet or inactive magnet (placebo) to the most sensitive sore spots of 50 subjects, who were experiencing arthritic or muscle pain. Overall,

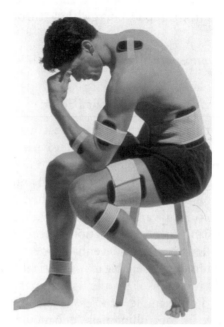

Figure 7-1   Pain has been the most emphasized magnetic-therapy application. (Photo provided by the FeelGood Company, Denver, CO.)

76% of the subjects who received the active magnet reported a decrease in pain. In contrast, only 19% with an inactive magnet felt an improvement. In another study, commercially available magnets were placed for one hour on the affected shoulder of eight subjects with SCI with myofascial shoulder pain. Results suggested that the magnets reduced this form of pain (4).

Spinal Cord Injury

Many scientists believe that electromagnetic energy will eventually play a paramount role in neuronal regeneration and restoring function after SCI. Animal and human studies indicate that pulsed electromagnetic fields stimulate both peripheral and spinal-cord neuronal regeneration, as well as functional recovery. These fields influence, for example, (a) calcium influx through the neuronal cell membrane, which affects essential cellular functions (5); (b) levels of key regeneration-affecting, nerve-growth factors (6); (c) the physical matrix of the tissue scar that forms after injury in a way that is less inhibitory to neuronal regrowth (7).

SCI clinical applications of magnetism are growing, including functional magnetic stimulation of urination and defecation, prevention of deep-vein thrombosis by inducing leg contractions, and increasing respiratory and coughing capability. In a recent pilot study, four patients with incomplete SCI had motor and sensory improvements after treatment with repetitive transcranial magnetic stimulation (rTMS), which generates brief magnetic pulses on the scalp. The investigators believe rTMS strengthens the information leaving the brain through the spinal cord's undamaged neurons (8). Another chapter will discuss how pulsed electromagnetic therapy promotes functional recovery after acute SCI and the healing of SCI-associated pressures sores.

Conclusions

Reflecting Paracelsus' statement "Magnetism is the king of all secrets," electromagnetism will most likely become a cornerstone of 21st century medicine. Its therapeutic potential already has more documented promise for SCI than most pharmaceutical and biochemical approaches that are the focus of the SCI-research establishment.

Additional Readings and Resources

Books

Lawrence R, Rosch PJ, Plowden J. *Magnetic Therapy: The Pain Cure Alternative.* Rocklin, Calif.: Prima Publishing, 1998.
Null G. *Healing with Magnets.* New York: Carroll & Graf, 1998.
Whitaker J, Adderly B. *The Pain Relief Breakthrough.* Boston: Little, Brown, 1998.
Payne B. *Magnetic Healing.* Twin Lakes, WI: Lotus Press, 1997.

PULSED ELECTROMAGNETIC THERAPY: DIAPULSE

This section of the chapter specifically discusses the use of Diapulse, a device that directs a pulsed-electromagnetic field (PEMF) to an area of injury. Animal and human studies indicate that this treatment administered soon after spinal cord injury (SCI) protects neurons, promotes regeneration, and minimizes lost function. In addition,

Diapulse greatly accelerates the healing of SCI-associated pressure sores.

Modern medicine focuses on the anatomical and biochemical (i.e., the physical), until recently ignoring the body's less understood electromagnetic nature. As underscored by Albert Einstein's $E = mc^2$ equation, however, the physical never exists without energy, and each influences the other. Every molecule in our body emits an electromagnetic field, and because each cell—and in turn each organ—is an aggregation of such molecules, they too are electromagnetic. There is no tissue in which this fact is more evident than our nervous system, which functions by routing electromagnetic impulses throughout our body via our spinal cord. Hence, attempts to fix an injured cord through physical means will be enhanced by working with and not against its electromagnetic nature.

Description

Diapulse directs electromagnetic energy to a specific body area, even through clothing, casts, or bandages, via a cylindrical treatment head that is mounted on an adjustable bracket (Figure 7-2). The

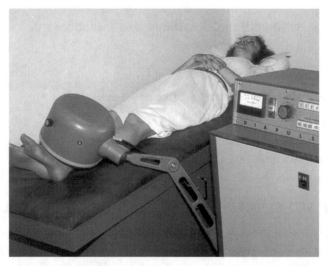

Figure 7-2   Diapulse directs electromagnetic energy to a specific body area via a cylindrical treatment head mounted on an adjustable bracket. (Photo provided by Diapulse Corporation.)

technology does not cause side effects or require patient involve-ment. Because the device pulses its electromagnetic output, it emits energy for only a fraction of time, allowing any heat associated with the transferred energy to dissipate. Diapulse's electromagnetic output is often 600 pulses per second, with each pulse lasting 65 microseconds (1 second = 1 million microseconds). Hence, this pulse rate corresponds to the device being off 25 times longer than it is on.

History

The Diapulse prototype was developed in the early 1930s by physi-cian Abraham Ginsberg and physicist Arthur Milinowski, who reported their initial clinical experience and animal research with the device to the 1934 and 1940 New York Academy of Medicine. Because the technology behind the device was used to develop radar, the device's emergence as a healing modality was delayed because of World War II security concerns.

Research was resumed in the 1950s by the military's Tri-Service Research Program, which after extensive studies concluded that the device was safe and effective. At about this time, the driving force behind Diapulse shifted from Ginsburg to Dr. Jesse Ross, a biophysi-cist, whose background includes professional associations with Ein-stein, and being one of the founders of the Bioelectromagnetic Society and a NASA consultant. Ross created the Diapulse Corpora-tion of America in Great Neck, New York, developing a collabora-tion with Remington Rand to produce the device. To further assess the device's healing potential, Ross then launched ambitious research with universities and clinicians around the world. Over time, Diapulse was adopted as a treatment in various areas of medi-cine throughout the world; in this country, it is approved by the FDA for treatment of postoperative swelling and pain.

Diapulse Studies

Numerous studies support Diapulse's potential to treat neurologi-cally associated problems and exert neuro-protective and -regenera-tive influences. After nervous-system injury, Diapulse helps to restore the membrane potential (the difference in concentration of charged solutes between the cell inside and outside) necessary to ensure cell survival and to enhance recovery-promoting blood flow.

Blood Flow

Dr. William Erdman of Philadelphia demonstrated that Diapulse increases systemic blood flow without elevating pulse rate or blood pressure (9). This effect most likely is because of the ability of Diapulse-generated fields to induce cells to align in a pearl-chain fashion. When the device was turned off, the cells reassumed a random distribution. With such an alignment, blood cells can more efficiently pass through a given vascular space, like cars traveling in the same direction on parallel lanes instead of like bumper cars.

As in all injuries, the rate of blood flow affects recovery after SCI. Specifically, the injury to the cord compromises blood flow, which consequently aggravates neurological damage. In a 2002 SCI conference, Dr. Henry Crock, a preeminent British authority on spinal cord circulation, stressed that blood flow is the primary factor that needs to be addressed after SCI (10). Given Diapulse's ability to enhance blood flow, it is not surprising that the device promotes healing after SCI.

Animal Studies

The first scientists to focus on Diapulse's neuronal regeneration properties were doctors D. Wilson and P. Jagadeesh of England (11). After demonstrating that the device stimulates regeneration in rats with peripheral nerve injuries (i.e., those outside the brain and spinal cord), they examined its effects on cats whose spinal cords were half cut (hemicordotomy). Compared to controls, three months after hemicordotomy, Diapulse improved functional recovery, reduced scar formation and adhesions, increased the number of axons transversing the injury site, and promoted the integration of peripheral nerve grafts that had been inserted to bridge the lesion. Doctors A. Raji and R. Bowden of London also demonstrated that Diapulse enhances regeneration and remyelination of rat peripheral nerves after transection (12).

Because surgeons are beginning to use peripheral nerve tissue to bridge spinal cord lesions in humans, Diapulse's ability to accelerate regeneration in peripheral tissue also has important therapeutic implications for SCI. Dr. Wise Young of New York showed that Diapulse reduces calcium at the injury site in cats injured through impact (an injury that resembles most human SCI). Because calcium causes secondary neuronal cell death, this Diapulse-induced reduction lessened neurological damage, and in turn preserved function (13–15). Specifically, Young reported that (a) the majority of cats treated by Diapulse were walking four months after surgery compared to none in the control group, and (b) the device was superior to treatment with the steroid methylprednisolone, now considered a postinjury treatment standard.

SCI Human Studies

Dr. Marion Weiss et al., of Warsaw, Poland, carried out a promising SCI study in 1980. Weiss, who received research funding from the U.S. Veterans Administration, arranged for acutely injured patients to be picked up by helicopter and brought to Warsaw where they were treated with Diapulse. Of the 97 treated patients, 38 had pronounced neurological improvement; of these, 28 had substantial functional gains, and 18 were discharged with only slight impairment of the extremities (16). Although this preliminary study lacked controls, these are impressive statistics, which, at minimum, warrant study replication. Unfortunately, because Weiss died soon after publishing these initial results, combined with post–Cold War social upheaval, this promising research was not continued.

Dr. W. Ellis anecdotally noted that PEMF given for pain in patients with chronic SCI resulted in sensory or motor improvement in 7 of 13 patients (17). Ellis hypothesized that these fields can normalize viable but dysfunctional neuronal structures. Finally, Diapulse therapy was recently used in Lisbon in conjunction with a function-restoring surgery in which olfactory tissue was transplanted into the SCI injury site. Specifically, Jesse Ross treated two Americans with quadriplegia with Diapulse several days before and after surgery to promote neuronal regeneration. Although it is difficult to sort out the relative contributions of the surgery, postsurgical rehabilitation, or Diapulse therapy, one of the patients had so much functional recovery that she was featured on a PBS documentary.

Pressure Sores

A number of studies demonstrate that Diapulse treatment greatly accelerates the healing of pressure sores (18–20), a serious SCI-associated problem, the complications of which caused the death of actor Christopher Reeve. In a specific SCI-focused, double-blind study, Dr. C. A. Salzberg et al. (Valhalla, New York) showed that the pressure sores of Diapulse-treated patients with SCI healed on average in 13 days compared to 31.5 days for controls (20).

Anna's Story

My husband is a T-8 paraplegic. He developed a severe decubitus ulcer of the coccyx, and it progressed to stage 4 (i.e., into the bone). Although he had home health care for almost three years, the wound continued. Health-care professionals took the approach of packing and probing with no success. Finally, a new wound-care specialist took time to do a lot of research and came up with the idea of using Diapulse therapy. Medicare refused to fund the cost, but our supplement paid the cost for eight weeks. The wound was about four centimeters deep and quite large in diameter. It was absolutely amazing—after eight weeks of four-times-a-day therapy, the wound healed completely. It is indeed a miracle cure for bedsores! (personal communication, July 18, 2003)

Conclusions

In addition to being a proven therapy for healing SCI-associated pressure sores, compelling evidence indicates that Diapulse-generated pulsed electromagnetic fields exert neuro-protective and -regenerative influences when administered soon after SCI. True SCI therapeutic potential still needs to be determined; however, given the amount of positive preliminary evidence, if Diapulse represented a more familiar pharmaceutical approach, the biomedical research community would be elated and would be pushing it to the forefront for further scrutiny instead of letting it languish.

FERRITE-RING MAGNETS

Compared to pulsed electromagnetic fields, ferrite-ring magnets represent a low-tech approach that may enhance functioning after spinal cord injury (SCI) and dysfunction (Figure 7-3). Ferrite ring magnets create a relatively powerful, toroidal spinning field, which in shape resembles the earth's magnetic field. Such a field more readily resonates with nature and living things. In a simple, yet

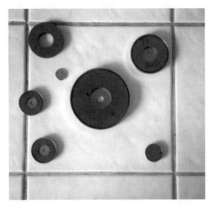

Figure 7-3   Ferrite-ring magnets of various sizes next to quarter for size comparison. (Photo taken by Laurance Johnston.)

visual, demonstration of field strength, a five-inch ring magnet is able to alter a television image from nearly two feet away. Clearly, these magnets have the potential to influence organs and physiology deep beneath the body's surface.

Because many commercially available products use relatively weak magnets, their effectiveness is questionable. For example, the magnets in many mattress pads are so weak that little field extends beyond the intervening padding, sheets, and pajamas.

The powerful ferrite ring magnets are inserted into various clothing or devices that place the magnets as close as possible to specific body areas. For example, in SCI, one could wear (or drape over a wheelchair back) a magnet-containing vest, sit over a magnet located under the wheelchair's seat cushion, and sleep on a mattress pad containing the ring magnets.

Case Examples

Lee, 29, was paralyzed in a construction accident. After a spinal-cord blood vessel burst, he progressively lost function, including bowel and bladder control and sexual ability, and could only walk a limited distance using a walker. Five months after injury, Lee started treatment with the ring magnets and obtained remarkable results. After a half year of therapy, Lee regained most of his lost function. Although I did not talk to Lee personally, a physician independently confirmed his recovery.

However, I did talk to Art and to Grace. Art became a C5-6 quadri-plegic in a 1981 car accident. His case represents an example of the more subtle improvement that may result from magnetic therapy many years after injury. A sports writer who recently obtained his Master's degree in rehabilitation counseling, Art has used ring magnets for four years and believes he has accrued subtle but significant benefits from them. He feels stronger, especially in the trunk region, has new tingling sensations that seem to grow with time, and sweats more than he has since his injury nearly 20 years ago. Furthermore, MRI imaging now indicates a much more viable spinal cord.

Grace, who has spina bifida (a neural tube birth defect in which a portion of the spinal cord protrudes through the vertebral column), had been plagued with recurring pressure sores. When her last sore would not heal, she tried the magnets. Because it was the first sore that healed without surgery, she is now a believer. What amazed Grace further were some other improvements that seemed to be correlated with her mag-netic therapy. Specifically, she could contract her left gluteal and thigh muscles for the first time, which she believes is indicative of some nerve healing. In addition, her left leg got longer with new bone growth as doc-umented by x-rays.

Conclusions

Because these represent a limited number of anecdotal cases with unique circumstances, we must be careful in extrapolating the results. Although dramatic results are probably the exception, subtle improvements that can significantly affect quality of life and inde-pendence may be a real possibility with perseverance.

Sources

With some research, including the Internet, ferrite-ring magnets can be obtained from numerous sources.

REFERENCES

1. Lawrence R, Rosch PJ, Plowden J. *Magnetic Therapy: The Pain Cure Alterna-tive*. Rocklin, Calif.: Prima Publishing, 1998.
2. Null G. *Healing with Magnets*. New York: Carroll and Graf, 1998.
3. Vallbona C, Hazlewood CF, Jurida G., Response of pain to static magnetic fields in postpolio patients: a double-blind pilot study. *Arch Phys Med Rehabil* 1997; 78: 1200–1203.

4. Panagos A, Jensen M, Cardenas DD. Treatment of myofascial shoulder pain in the spinal cord injured population using static magnetic fields: a case series. *J Spinal Cord Med* 2004; 27: 138–142.

5. Young W. Pulsed electromagnetic fields alter calcium in spinal cord injury. *The 75th Meeting of the Society of Neurological Surgeons*, New York, April 25–28, 1984.

6. Longo FM, Yang T, Hamilton S, et al. Electromagnetic fields influence NGF activity and levels following sciatic nerve transection. *J Neurosci Res* 1999; 55: 230–237.

7. Tkach EV, Abilova AN, Gazalieva SM. Characteristics of the effect of a constant electromagnetic field on reparative processes in spinal cord injuries. *Zh Nevropatol Psikhiatr Im S S Korsakova* 1989; 89(5): 41–44.

8. Belci M, Catley M, Husain M, et al. Magnetic brain stimulation can improve clinical outcome in incomplete spinal cord injured patients. *Spinal Cord* 2004; 42: 417–419.

9. Erdman WJ. Peripheral blood flow measurements during application of pulsed high frequency currents, *Am J Ortho* 1960; 2: 196–197.

10. Johnston L. Promising procedures: world-renowned scientists share a stimulating exchange that indicates hope for the future of SCI research. *Paraplegia News* 2002; 56(8): 15–17.

11. Wilson DH, Jagadeesh P. Experimental regeneration in peripheral nerves and the spinal cord in laboratory animals exposed to a pulsed electromagnetic field. *Paraplegia* 1976; 14: 12–20.

12. Raji ARM, Bowden REM. Effects of high-peak pulsed electromagnetic field on the degeneration and regeneration of the common peroneal nerve in rats. *J Bone and Joint Surg* 1983; 65B(4): 478–492.

13. Young W, Koreh I, Ransohoff J. Pulsed electromagnetic fields alter tissue calcium accumulation, *Presentation to American Paralysis Association 1983 Workshop*.

14. Young W. Pulsed electromagnetic fields alter calcium in spinal cord injury. *Presentation to the 75th Meeting of the Society of Neurological Surgeons*, New York, April 25–28, 1984.

15. Young W. Pulsed electromagnetic fields (Diapulse) alter calcium in spinal cord injury, *Presentation to American Paralysis Association Meeting*, San Francisco, May 20, 1984.

16. Kiwerski J, Chrostowska T, Weiss M. Clinical trials of the application of pulsating electromagnetic energy (Diapulse) in the treatment of spinal cord lesions. *Narz Ortoped, Pol* 1980; 45: 273–277.

17. Ellis W. Pulsed subcutaneous electrical stimulation in spinal cord injury. *Bioelectromagnetics* 1987; 8: 159–164.

18. Itoh M, Montemayor JS, Matsumoto E, et al. Accelerated wound healing of pressure ulcers by pulsed high peak power electromagnetic energy (Diapulse). *Decubitus* 1994; 4(1): 24–34.

19. Comorsan S, Vasilco R, Arhiroplo M, et al. The effects of Diapulse therapy on the healing of decubitus sores. *Romanian J Phys (Physiological Sciences)* 1993; 30 (1–2): 41–45.

20. Salzberg CA, Cooper-Vastola SA, Perez FJ, et al. The effects of non-thermal pulsed electromagnetic energy (Diapulse) on wound healing of pressure ulcers in spinal cord-injured patients: a randomized, double-blind study. *Wounds* 1995; 7(1): 11–16.

8

Indigenous Healing

NATIVE-AMERICAN HEALING: PART 1—PHILOSOPHY

In my efforts to expand the healing spectrum of individuals with spinal cord injury (SCI), I have reviewed diverse healing approaches, none of which has been more intriguing yet initially alien to my Western-trained scientific mind than Native-American medicine. As a scientist who uses physical laws to dissect the microcosm further, I was challenged to absorb metaphorically the spiritual, cosmological, and ecological views of the macrocosm that shape Native-American healing.

In *The Way of the Scout: A Native American Path to Finding Spiritual Meaning in a Physical World* (1), Tom Brown, Jr. describes how when he was a child an Apache elder taught him to use an "expanded focus," where the task (i.e., any of life's pursuits) is but a small part of the whole picture. When we relax an absolute focus, we become more aware of life's flow around us, and as a result, assistance in many unanticipated forms becomes available. For most of us who view the world through the conditioning of Western thought, an expanded focus fosters a greater understanding of Native-American wisdom. In my case, as I relaxed the rigidity of my scientific beliefs, an understanding grew that complemented, not negated, these beliefs.

Contributions

Throughout our nation's history, Native-American societal contributions have been immense but often unrecognized. A few examples include Benjamin Franklin's modeling the Articles of Confederation on the Iroquois nation's constitution, World War II's Navajo code breakers, tribal donations of more than $200,000 for post–9/11 relief efforts, and the first servicewoman killed in Iraq being a Hopi Indian. Furthermore, much of the world's foods and medicines have Native-American origins (2). For example, more than 200 Native-American herbal medicines have been listed at one time or another in the U.S. Pharmacopoeia; many modern drugs have botanical origins in these medicines.

Indigenous Medicine

Native-American medicine is classified as an indigenous healing tradition. Because 80% of the world's population cannot afford Western high-tech medicine, indigenous traditions collectively play an important role in global health care role, so much so that the World Health Organization recommended that they be integrated into national health-care policies and programs. Although Native-American healing reflects the diversity of the many Native nations or tribes that have inhabited "Turtle Island" (i.e., North America), common themes exist not only between them but with many of the world's geographically diverse, ancient indigenous traditions.

The Role of Spirit and Connection

A major difference between Native-American and conventional medicine concerns the role of spirit and connection. Although spirituality has been a key component of healing through most of humankind's history, modern medicine eschews it, embracing a mechanistic view that the body is fixable pursuant to physical laws of science.

In contrast, Native-American medicine considers spirit, whose life-force manifestation in humans is called *ni* by the Lakota and *nilch'i* by the Navajo, an inseparable element of healing (3). Not only is the patient's spirit important but also the spirit of the healer, the patient's family, community, and environment, and the medicine itself. More important, healing must take into account the dynamics between these spiritual forces as a part of the universal spirit.

Instead of modern medicine's view of separation that focuses on fixing unique body parts in distinct individuals separate from each other and the environment, Native Americans believe we are all synergistically part of a whole that is greater than the sum of the parts; healing must be considered within this context. Specifically, we are all connected at some level to each other, Mother Earth (nature), Father Sky, and all of life through the *Creator* (Iroquois), *Great Spirit* (Lakota), *Great Mystery* (Ojibway), or *Maker of All Things Above* (Crow) (3). This sense of wholeness and connection is implied by the concluding phrase of healing prayers and chants "All my Relations," which dedicates these invocations to all physical and spiritual relations that are a part of the Great Spirit (3). To describe our universal connection metaphorically, the Lakota use the phrase *mitakuye oyasin*—"We are all related"—whereas Pueblo tribes of the Southwest, who consider corn as a life symbol, say "We are all kernels on the same corncob" (2).

In *Native Science: Natural Laws of Interdependence* (2), Dr. Gregory Cajete uses modern science's chaos theory to support the Native-American concept of connection. Sometimes called the butterfly effect, this theory postulates that the flapping of a butterfly's wing may initiate a disturbance that ultimately leads to a hurricane or another phenomenon across the world. Whether it is this wing-flapping, a prayer for healing, or one's stand against oppression, chaos theory, as well as Native-American philosophy, implies that everything is related and has an influence no matter how small. Moreover, we all have "butterfly power" to create from the inherent chaos of our universe, which Cajete describes as "not simply a collection of objects, but rather a dynamic, ever-flowing river of creation inseparable from our own perceptions" (p. 15).

Cultural Rebirth

Although you cannot appreciate Native-American medicine without its spiritual dynamics, the practice of Native-American spirituality surprisingly was banned in this land of religious freedom until the 1978 passage of the American Indian Religious Freedom Act. For example, in *Coyote Medicine: Lessons from Native American Healing* (4), Dr. Lewis Mehl-Madrona tells how he risked jail by attending an early 1970s healing ceremony. Because of this ban, which forbade congregating and keeping sacred objects, much of Native-American healing was driven underground or to extinction. It is the equivalent of telling physicians they can't practice medicine if they do surgeries or prescribe drugs. Since the prohibition's lifting, however, worldwide interest in Native-American wisdom has soared, in part because

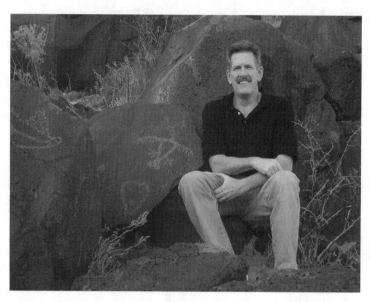

Figure 8-1 The author next to a petroglyph of "Thunderbird," a mythological being who speaks in thunder and lightening and teaches us how to use its power to heal. Because it is a symbol for our body's electrical current, Thunderbird is invoked by Native-American healers for nervous-system disorders. (Photo taken by Doug Crispin.)

it is perceived as an antidote to modern society's soul-depleting and environment-damaging aspects.

Disability

The idea of wholeness is paramount in understanding Native-American perception of disability. Unlike many cultures that shun people with disabilities, Native Americans honor and respect them. They believe that a person weak in body is often blessed by the Creator by being especially strong in mind and spirit. By reducing our emphasis on the physical, which promotes our view of separation from other human beings and all that is, a greater sense of connection with the whole is created, the ultimate source of strength. Overall, in treating physical disability, Native-American healers emphasize quality of life, getting more in touch with and honoring inherent gifts, adjusting one's mind-set, and learning new tools. By so doing, the individual's humanity is optimized.

Distinguishing Features

In addition to these overarching philosophical differences, there are many other features that distinguish Native-American from Western medicine. In *Honoring the Medicine: The Essential Guide to Native American Healing* (4), recently selected as the National Multiple Sclerosis Society's Wellness Book of the Year, Kenneth "Bear Hawk" Cohen summarizes some of theses features in a table (see Table 8-1, abstracted with permission from the author).

Additional Readings and Resources

See *Readings and Resources* at the end of part 2 of this chapter.

Table 8.1 Distinguishing Features Between Western and Native-American Medicine

WESTERN MEDICINE	NATIVE-AMERICAN MEDICINE
Focus on pathology and curing disease	Focus on health and healing the person and community
Reductionistic: Diseases are biological, and treatment should produce measurable outcomes.	*Complex:* Diseases do not have a simple explanation, and outcomes are not always measurable.
Adversarial medicine: "How can I destroy the disease?"	*Teleological medicine:* "What can the disease teach the patient? Is there a message or story in the disease?"
Investigate disease with a "divide-and-conquer" strategy, looking for microscopic cause.	Looks at the "big picture": the causes and effects of disease in the physical, emotional, environmental, social, and spiritual realms
Intellect is primary. Medical practice is based on scientific theory.	Intuition is primary. Healing is based on spiritual truths learned from nature, elders, and spiritual vision.
Physician is an authority.	Healer is a health counselor and advisor.
Fosters dependence on medication, technology	Empowers patients with confidence, awareness, and tools to help them take charge of their own health.
Health history focuses on patient and family: "Did your mother have cancer?"	Health history includes the environment: "Are the salmon in your rivers ill?"
Intervention should result in rapid cure or management of disease.	Patience is paramount. Healing occurs when the time is right.

NATIVE-AMERICAN HEALING:
PART 2–HEALING MODALITIES

Part 1 discussed key characteristics of Native-American medicine. It focused on the paramount role of spirit, including not only in the patient but also the healer, family, community, environment, and medicine, and the dynamics between these forces as a part of the Universal Spirit.

Part 2 summarizes specific healing modalities, some of which can be understood, at least superficially, through conventional biological mechanisms (e.g., herbal remedies) and others that must be understood, once again, within a greater spiritual context. Basically, the fundamental goal of all Native-American healing is to establish a better spiritual equilibrium between patients and their universe, which in turn translates into physical and mental health.

Medicine Is Spirit

Marilyn Youngbird (of the Arikara and Hidatsa nations), an international lecturer on native wisdom and former Colorado Commissioner for Indian Affairs, emphasized Spirit's overriding role to me:

> It is difficult for the average American, who thinks medicine is merely swallowing a pill, to understand that medicine does not live outside of us. Medicine is a part of Spirit that exists in, animates, and connects all of us. Spirit is *life*, and its healing energy is available to us if we learn to know, live, breathe, walk, and speak it.

Native-American Disability

Eighteenth-century records suggest that paralysis was rare among Native Americans before contact with Whites. Today, however, their SCI incidence is two to four times that of Whites because they face more of modern society's injury-aggravating downside (primarily mediated through motor vehicle accidents) combined with the historical suppression of mitigating cultural support systems.

Native Americans traditionally believed that a person weak in body is strong in mind and spirit. According to *The Native Americans* (5), such conviction is "related to the all-pervasive regard for differences . . . the curtailing of some ability, whether physical or mental, was more than compensated for by some special gift at storytelling, herbal cures, tool-making, oratory, or putting people at ease" (p. 118). Traditionally, Native Americans thought that many inherited disorders were caused by parents' unhealthy or immoral behavior (fetal alcohol syndrome would be a good example in today's world) (3). The Delaware and other tribes believed paralysis resulted from a patient's or parent's breach of taboo, and the Comanche called it a "ghost sickness" created by negative spirits or sorcery. Because it was thought that some diseases or disorders were the result of the patient's behavior, it was believed that treatment might interfere with important life lessons.

Approaches to Healing

Because it is difficult to summarize succinctly a subject as involved as Native-American medicine and do it justice, interested readers are encouraged to review *Honoring the Medicine* (4) by Kenneth "Bear Hawk" Cohen (who was adopted by the Cree nation), selected as the National MS Society Wellness Book of the Year.

Plants

Because of Native Americans' intimate relationship with nature, many therapies emphasize plants' mind–body–spirit healing potential.

Herbs

Native-American herbalism is much more complex than herbs merely serving as a plant matrix to deliver physiologically active chemicals (3, 4). First, because numerous plant components affect bodily functions and bioavailability, the entire remedy is considered the active agent. Second, because plants are believed to possess spirit and intelligence, they are consulted to determine their best healing relationship with patients, and permission is obtained before, and gratitude expressed after, harvesting them. Third, intricate procedures are used to harvest herbs, considering factors such as plant part (e.g., flower, stem, root, etc.), time or season of harvesting, sun exposure, and other much more obscure factors. Fourth, native herbalists use plants that appear in dreams, a form of communication by which the plant's spirit can guide the healer. Finally, the plant's healing potential is empowered by ritual ceremony, prayer, song, or chants. Cohen notes that although herbs can treat symptoms without such empowerment, they will not reach the deeper causes of illness.

Tobacco

Ironically, the most spiritually powerful plant is tobacco (3, 4), modern society's substance of greatest abuse. Tobacco is the herb of prayer, placed on earth by spirits to help us communicate with them and nature. All tobacco use, ranging from ceremonial to cigarettes, should be treated with respect and awareness. Specifically, the famous elder Rolling Thunder (a Cherokee) taught Cohen the following:

> After you light tobacco, with your first puff, you should think a good thought or make a prayer. With your second, quiet your mind; rest in stillness. With your third puff, you can receive insight related to your prayer—perhaps an image, words spoken by spirit, or an intuitive feeling.

Smudge

Other sacred plants are used for smudging, a purification procedure in which a plant's aromatic smoke cleanses an area of negative energies, thoughts, feelings, and spirits (3, 4) (Figure 8-2). Smudging is a key component of healing prayers and ceremonies. The most commonly used plants are sage (not the spice) and cedar, which drive out negative energy; and sweetgrass, which invites in positive, healing spirits. Cohen believes that all healers should smudge between clients to prevent the transfer of pathogenic energy.

Prayer, Chants, and Music

Prayer is pervasive in Native-American healing. As reviewed elsewhere in this book, substantial scientific evidence exists that prayer can affect health. As Cohen notes, Native-American prayer concentrates the mind on healing, promotes health-enhancing emotions and feelings, and connects people to sacred healing forces (3, 4). In contrast to more familiar whispered prayers, Native Americans robustly proclaim, chant, or sing prayers. Singing is often accompanied by drumming or rattles, which, by synchronizing group consciousness, greatly magnifies healing impact.

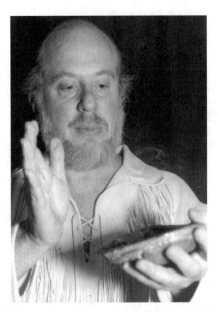

Figure 8-2 Smudging is a purification procedure in which a plant's aromatic smoke cleanses an area of negative energies, thoughts, feelings, and spirits. (Photo provided by Kenneth Cohen.)

Lewis Mehl-Madrona (a Cherokee), an emergency-room physician and author of *Coyote Medicine* (6), told me that prayer should be incorporated into overall therapy after any major injury: "At the time of acute injury, enroll everyone—patient, family members, friends, doctors, nurses—in a prayer circle with the expectation of the best outcome."

Therapeutic Touch and Energy Work

Native-American medicine includes many approaches with similarities to today's alternative bodywork or energy-related techniques, including massage, therapeutic touch, and acupressure-like stimulation of body points (3, 4).

Counseling

Counseling helps patients find a more health-promoting, mind–body–spirit balance through, for example, developing a better understanding of a life path and purpose or the role that the disease or disorder plays. Because the counseling is based on spiritual wisdom, Cohen likens it more to pastoral counseling than to psychotherapy (3, 4).

Ceremony

Native-American ceremonies incorporate a variety of healing modalities into a ritualized context for seeking spiritual guidance (3, 4). According to Cohen, one of the ceremony's chief goals is communicating with the spirit of a disease to gather information that can lead to the release of pathogenic forces. Mehl-Madrona indicated to me that "at one time in their history, all cultures have had beneficial healing ceremonies; unfortunately, most modern, white-culture ceremonies have become so sterile they are not conducive for healing."

I participated in a sweat-lodge ceremony in the traditional Lakota style. It was held in a dome-like structure covered by tarps and heated by pouring water over hot stones (the stone people). Tobacco prayer ties were hung inside, smudging herbs sprinkled on the stones, and sacred pipes ceremonially smoked. Participants prayed, sang, and chanted to obtain guidance, wisdom, and healing not only for themselves but for all who are a part of Mother Earth's greater unity. Overall, the sweat-lodge's mind–body–spirit purification, communion-with-spirit process helps people understand who they are, especially relative to any disease or disorder. With such empowering understanding, you start reclaiming responsibility for and taking charge of your own soul rather than relinquishing its direction to health-care authorities.

Because the sweat lodge is totally dark except for the faint glow of hot stones, no one has a disability in the ceremony; everyone is an equal participant. The ceremony can target underlying emotional causes of substance abuse, a problem that plagues many with SCI. It can also promote healing at different levels by generating forgiveness, releasing bitterness, and busting apart the self-fulfilling belief pattern—which is imprinted onto most patients after an injury—that they will never walk again. (Because the sweat lodge is indeed hot, it is not recommended for those with higher level, sweat-inhibiting injuries.)

Mehl-Madrona developed a program based on Native-American values and beliefs that emphasizes ceremony and targets non-natives who have chronic disease or disorders (6). Mehl-Madrona

reported that more than 80% of program enrollees accrued significant, persistent benefits.

A Case Study

The following case study, involving not SCI but another form of
spinal cord dysfunction, illustrates many of the previously discussed
approaches. Specifically, Cohen used Si Si Wiss healing—an inter-
tribal tradition from the Puget Sound area—to restore ambulatory
function in Jon, an Icelandic man with multiple sclerosis (MS).

Because of chronic knee pain, Jon could not place his full weight on his
left leg and could only walk short distances using a walker (7). Cohen
believes that location played a key role in Jon's healing. Native Americans believe that certain geographical locations possess strong healing
energy (among Christians, the most well-known such site is Lourdes,
France). Cohen was lecturing near Iceland's Snæfellsnes Glacier, a legend-
ary Nordic sacred area that author Jules Verne chose for his intrepid
explorers to start their descent in *Journey to the Center of the Earth*.
From his audience, Cohen recruited participants for a healing circle that
surrounded Jon and instructed them to sing a healing song to a drum
beat.
     Cohen relates the incidents this way:

> I cleansed Jon with a smudge of local bearberry leaves and juniper.
> As I waved the smoke around his body with my hands, I also imag-
> ined that Grandmother Ocean (within view) was purifying him. I
> then placed my hands on Jon's spine, one palm at his sacrum, the
> other above his seventh cervical vertebrae. I rested my palms there
> for a few minutes, to both "read" the energy in his spine and to
> focus healing and loving power.
>   I then held his knee lightly between my two palms, focusing
> with the same intent. After this, I did noncontact treatment, primar-
> ily over Jon's head, focusing on the brain itself. I held my hands a
> few inches from his skull, one hand in front, one in back, then one
> hand to the left, one to the right. I continued, holding my palms
> above his spine, moving them gently up from the sacrum towards
> the crown and then down the front midline of his body.
>   As I continued with noncontact treatment, I prayed in a soft
> voice, yet loud enough for Jon to hear me, and with a tone, rhythm,
> and intensity that harmonized with the sound of the background
> singing and drumming. "Oh Creator, I ask for healing for this
> brother. Let him learn his lessons through your guidance and
> wisdom, not through pain. I pray that whether this condition
> was caused by inner or outside forces, whether originating from

this time or any time in the past, whether intentionally caused by offended people or spirits or caused by chance—let the pain and disability be lifted and released in a good and natural way.

At the ceremony's end, I helped him to stand and was about to move his walker over to him, when he said, "No, wait a moment. I feel something." He began to walk without assistance, slowly but with an apparently normal gait. He showed no sign of unsteadiness and was able to use his left leg easily. I walked alongside of Jon, expecting him to lose balance and fall. Instead, he turned towards me, embraced me and said, tearfully, "Thank God! It's a miracle. I can walk!"

Residents of Jon's village, who had known him for many years, later expressed their amazement to Cohen of seeing Jon walking about town normally.

Cohen's treatment included therapeutic energy work. As such, it should be noted that his ability to transfer electromagnetic energy through intention, with and without direct touch, has been documented in rigorous experiments at the prestigious Menninger Clinic. In fact, because of Cohen's reputation, many of his patients have been referred to him by physicians.

Conclusions

The study of Native American and other indigenous healing traditions is important because they have greatly influenced modern medicine in spite of major philosophical differences; collectively still play a huge role in global health care; and offer solutions to modern society's ailments that spiritually bereft science cannot. Native Americans believe their actions must consider the welfare of the seventh generation to come. Perhaps this is why their ancient wisdom is not just intriguing anthropological residuum pushed aside by Western civilization, but is reemerging in relevance to the present generation.

Acknowledgment

The author expresses gratitude for all his teachers of native wisdom, especially Kenneth Cohen.

Additional Readings and Resources

Books

Ballantine B, Ballantine I, eds. *The Native Americans: An Illustrated History.* North Dighton, Mass.: JG Press, 2001.

Boyd D. *Rolling Thunder: A Personal Exploration into the Secret Healing Powers of an American Indian Medicine Man.* New York: Random House, 1974.

Brown T Jr. *Grandfather: A Native American's Lifelong Search for Truth and Harmony with Nature.* New York: Berkley Books, 1993.

Brown T Jr. *The Way of the Scout: A Native American Path to Finding Spiritual Meaning in a Physical World.* New York: Berkley Books, 1995.

Cajete G. *Native Science: Natural Laws of Interdependence.* Santa Fe, NM: Clear Light Publishers, 2000.

Cohen K. *Honoring the Medicine: The Essential Guide to Native American Healing.* New York: One World Ballantine Books, 2003.

Garrett JT, Garrett M. *Medicine of the Cherokee: The Way of Right Relationship.* Santa Fe, NM: Bear and Company, 1996.

Kavash EB, Baar K. *American Indian Healing Arts: Herbs, Rituals, and Remedies for Every Season of Life.* New York: Bantam Books, 1999.

Lux MK. *Medicine That Walks: Disease, Medicine, and Canadian Plains Native People, 1880–1940.* Toronto: University of Toronto Press, 2001.

Mails TE. *The Hopi Survival Kit,* New York: Welcome Rain, 1997.

Mehl-Madrona L. *Coyote Medicine: Lessons from Native American Healing.* New York: Simon and Schuster, 1997.

Neihardt JG. *Black Elk Speaks.* New York: Simon and Schuster, 1972.

Nerburn K. *The Wisdom of the Native Americans.* Novato, Calif.: New World Library, 1999.

Null G. *Secrets of the Sacred White Buffalo: Native American Healing Remedies, Rites, and Rituals.* Paramus, NJ: Prentice-Hall, 1998.

Rhoades ER, ed. *American Indian Health: Innovations in Health Care, Promotion, and Policy.* Baltimore, Md.: Johns Hopkins University Press, 2000.

Villoldo A. *Shaman, Healer, Sage: How to Heal Yourself and Others with the Energy Medicine of the Americas.* New York: Harmony Books, 2000.

Journals

Cohen K. Native American medicine. *Alternative Therapies,* 1998; 4(6):45–57.

Mehl-Madrona L. Native American medicine in the treatment of chronic illness: developing an integrated program and evaluating its effectiveness. *Alternative Therapies,* 1999; 5(1):36–44.

REFERENCES

1. Brown T Jr. *The Way of the Scout: A Native American Path to Finding Spiritual Meaning in a Physical World.* New York: Berkley Books, 1995.

2. Cajete G. *Native Science: Natural Laws of Interdependence*. Santa Fe, NM: Clear Light Publishers, 2000.
3. Cohen K. Native American Medicine. *Alternative Therapies*, 1998; 4(6): 45–57.
4. Cohen K. *Honoring the Medicine: The Essential Guide to Native American Healing*. New York: One World Ballantine Books, 2003.
5. Ballantine B, Ballantine I, eds. *The Native Americans: An Illustrated History*. North Dighton, Mass.: JG Press, 2001.
6. Mehl-Madrona L. Native American medicine in the treatment of chronic illness: developing an integrated program and evaluating its effectiveness. *Alternative Therapies*, 1999; 5(1):36–44.
7. Cohen K. American Indian healing in land of fire and ice: Available online at www.wholistichealingresearch.com

9

Prayer, Consciousness, Energy, and Spiritual Healing

PART 1:
SPIRITUALITY AND HEALTH

Many alternative therapies emphasize healing from a mind–body–spirit perspective. Mind–body approaches to medicine have gained increasing acceptance in recent years. What about spirituality? Almost everyone prays when faced with a traumatic injury like spinal cord injury (SCI) or serious disease. Can this prayer actually help? Substantial scientific evidence indicates that it can. This chapter will discuss some of the evidence correlating religion, spirituality, and prayer with physical health. Part 2 of this chapter will discusses several possible mechanisms by which spiritual healing or prayerlike consciousness can facilitate physical healing.

Prayer: A Medical Taboo?

Preferring drugs, surgery, and high technology, modern medicine has ignored healing's spiritual components. Physical laws delineated by Sir Isaac Newton in the 17th century guide modern medicine. Under these laws, the universe—including the human body—functions by specific cause-and-effect physical principles. As such, the body can be understood by breaking down and studying each component. Because consciousness plays no role in such a system, spirituality has been considered irrelevant to health.

In addition, many people are leery of scientists attempting to study prayer. They believe scientists' attitudes have contributed to many of the world's problems and do not want prayer debased by scientific scrutiny. Society has a tendency to compartmentalize prayer and spirituality. For example, the National Institutes of Health (NIH) was criticized for sponsoring a study examining the effect of prayer in alcohol and drug rehabilitation because it supposedly violated the separation of church and state (1). Because of such controversies and biases, many scientists prefer to use phrases like "subtle energy fields" when describing their research on prayerlike consciousness. Where prayer is thought of as possessing emotional, subjective connotations, subtle energy research is carried out by objective "hard" scientists. Nevertheless, many scientists have thought that science and spirituality enhance each other and do not represent incompatible views of the world. As Albert Einstein stated, "Science without religion is lame. Religion without science is blind."

The Comeback of Prayer

Prayer is making a medical comeback. Given that most Americans believe in God or a higher power (2), it is not surprising that 75% of patients think their physician should address spiritual issues as part of their medical care. Furthermore, 40% want their physicians to discuss religious issues actively with them, and nearly 50% percent want their physicians to pray not just *for* them but *with* them. In a growing trend, 43% of American physicians privately pray for their patients (1). An article in the *Journal of the American Medical Association* (2) entitled "Should Physicians Prescribe Prayer for Health?" discusses these trends. The mere presence of this article in this highly respected bastion of the medical profession suggests that the barrier between spirituality and health care is crumbling.

Organized Religion: Good for Your Health?

Scientific studies demonstrate that individuals who participate in organized religion are physically healthier and living longer (3). For example, they have lower blood pressure and incidence of stroke and heart disease. Regarding mental health, they have lower rates of depression, anxiety, substance abuse, and suicide. Organized religion can promote health through a variety of social mechanisms, for example, by discouraging unhealthy behaviors such as alcohol and drug use, smoking, and high-risk sex; and by providing social support and a sense of belonging.

The Science Behind Prayer

In addition to the effects of organized religion, prayerlike conscious-ness also has been shown to exert an influence in numerous scientific studies. Although the effects of organized religion can be explained through readily understandable mechanisms, the effects of prayer cannot. Dr. Daniel Benor has reviewed the scientific literature and found 131 controlled studies involving prayer or spiritual healing (4). Of these, 77 showed statistically significant results.

Lower Life Forms

Through conscious intent, test subjects (i.e., normal volunteers with no special abilities) were able to influence the growth of fungus, molds, yeast, and bacteria, often at great distances. These studies imply that prayer has the potential to fight infections (4, 5). With potentially profound implications, subjects were also able to alter the genetic mutation rate of bacteria.

DNA Expression

If prayer can alter the genetics of bacteria, it is conceivable that it could do so in humans also. If this is indeed the case, humans may not be limited to what was previously thought to be a genetic destiny they were born with. Author Gregg Braden believes that human emotion affects the patterning of the body's DNA (the genetic material) (6).

Dr. Bruce Lipton, a membrane biochemist, supports this belief and has hypothesized that our emotions affect our DNA patterning by influencing proteins embedded in our cell membranes (7). Specif-ically, he notes that (a) our emotions or conscious intent can alter our electromagnetic fields (see part 2 of this chapter) and (b) changes in such electromagnetic fields can affect the activity of membrane proteins that influence DNA expression within cells.

Human Studies

Prayerlike consciousness has been shown to inhibit the growth of cancer cells, protect red blood cells, alter blood chemistry, and increase blood oxygenation (4, 5). In one study, skin wounds healed at a much greater rate when treated with a spirituality-related treatment (perhaps an option for pressure sores).

In a paradigm-expanding study carried out by cardiologist Randolph Byrd, nearly 400 heart patients were randomly assigned either to a group that was prayed for by a home prayer group or a control group (8). This was a methodologically rigorous double-blind study designed to eliminate the psychological placebo effect. In such a study, neither the patient nor doctor knows who is receiving the intervention (in this case, prayer). Patients who received prayer had better health outcomes, including a reduced need for antibiotics and a lower incidence of pulmonary edema. Validating this study, the benefits of remote, intercessory prayer on health outcomes were later independently documented in a much larger double-blind study involving 990 cardiac patients (9).

Prayer's potential healing power was further demonstrated in a study carried out by Dr. Elizabeth Targ (10). In this study, advanced AIDS patients who received an hour of distant prayer six days a week for 10 weeks were significantly healthier than those who received no prayer. For example, patients who were prayed for required 85% fewer days of hospitalization, 29% fewer doctor visits, and developed 83% fewer new illnesses than the control group. The 40 individuals praying for patients represented seven different religious traditions.

Prayer researcher Jack Stucki has carried out double-blind studies evaluating the effects of distant prayer on the body's electromagnetic fields (personal communication, December 18, 1998). In these studies, the electrical activity in both the brain and body surface was measured in subjects in his Colorado Springs laboratory. Nearly 1,000 miles away in California, spiritual groups would either pray or not pray for a subject. The electrical activity measured in the subjects who were prayed for was significantly altered compared to controls.

As discussed in chapter 8, Native Americans believe that prayer should be incorporated into overall therapy after any major injury. Dr. Lewis Mehl-Madrona (a Cherokee), an emergency-room physician and author, states: "At the time of acute injury, enroll everyone—patient, family members, friends, doctors, nurses—in a prayer circle with the expectation of the best outcome" (personal communication, June 27, 2004). Given these and other studies, it would be theoretically relatively straightforward to design a study to determine whether group prayer would help minimize neurological damage after acute SCI. What do we have to lose except our paradigms?

Healing Through Secondary Materials

Spiritual healers have been shown to mediate healing through secondary materials, such as water or surgical gauze, which they have held (11, 12). A spectroscopic analysis of healer-treated water indicated an energy-induced shift in the water's molecular structure. This healer-treated water maintained these altered properties and its effectiveness for at least two years. These findings suggest that it is indeed possible for sacred objects, such as holy water, to possess power.

Nonlocal Prayer

The preceding examples indicate that prayer and spiritual healing can exert its effect from a distance. As discussed in Larry Dossey's *Healing Words* (5), test subjects (again, "normal" volunteers with no special gifts) can influence the outcome of random physical events even when separated by great distances. This research, much of which was carried out at Princeton University, uses random-event or number generators. These generators produce large sets of data like zeros and ones, which should average out over time as in the case of flipping a coin. Subjects, however, can influence the outcome of these generators so the data no longer average out (i.e., are no longer random).

Time-Displaced Prayer

Test subjects not only can influence outcomes over distance but, amazingly, can also affect past outcomes (5). Specifically, the subjects influenced the output of random-event generators *in the past*. In these cause-is-after-the-effect experiments, the random events have already been recorded but not consciously observed. This after-the-fact influencing was blocked, however, if another party (even an animal) observed the prerecorded data before the mental influence was attempted. Hence, conscious observation seems to fix the past.

If we can influence the past outcomes of random event generators, some of which are based on atomic decay, is it possible to influence our medical past, which is also based on atomic events? For example, although annual physical exams can uncover problems at an early stage, there is no statistical evidence that such exams increase longevity in the general population. Although being careful

not to encourage individuals to forgo such exams, Dr. Dossey speculates that the physical exam may serve as the act of observation that
irrevocably locks the disease in place. This "medical looking" may
"erase the malleability of critical physiological events" that many
individuals may have been able to influence at some mind–body–
spirit level if they had not been examined (5).

A New Energy?

Quantum physics is developing theories with insights into nonlocal
phenomena such as distant prayer (5). For example, Bell's theorem,
which is supported by experimental evidence, indicates that once
subatomic particles have been in contact, they always remain connected. A change in one creates a concurrent change in the other
even if they are a universe apart. Some physicists believe that these
nonlocal events are not just limited to subatomic particles but under-
lie everyday events, including prayer. To help understand a number
of inexplicable phenomena, including nonlocal events, many physicists believe that a fifth form of energy exists (in addition to gravity,
electromagnetic energy, and strong and weak nuclear energy) that
operates on different principles. Perhaps the life-force energy
referred to by many medical and spiritual traditions throughout
history represents this energy. Is it the energy referred to as prana
in India and Tibet, mana by the Polynesians, Yesad in the Jewish
Kabalistic tradition, qi in oriental medicine, or the Christian
Holy Spirit?

Additional Readings and Resources

Books

Benor DJ. *Healing Research: Holistic Energy Medicine and Spirituality Vol 1*. Dedding-
    ton, Oxfordshire, UK: Helix 1993.
Dossey L. *Healing Words: The Power of Prayer and the Practice of Medicine*. New
    York: HarperCollins, 1993.
Dossey L. *Prayer Is Good Medicine*. New York: HarperCollins Publishers, 1996.
Koenig HG. *Is Religion Good for Your Health?* Binghamton, NY: Haworth Press,
    1997.
Radin D. *The Conscious Universe*. New York: HarperCollins, 1997.
Targ R, Katra J. *Miracles of the Mind: Exploring Nonlocal Consciousness and Spiritual
    Healing*. Novato, Calif.: New World Library, 1999.

Weston W. *How Prayer Heals*. Charlottesville, Va.: Hampton Roads Publishing, 1998.

PART 2:
HOW SPIRITUALITY CAN PROMOTE PHYSICAL HEALING

Part 1 focused on how prayer, spirituality, and consciousness can influence health. Part 2 discusses several possible mechanisms, including electromagnetic ones, by which therapies based on prayer-like consciousness can facilitate physical healing.

Electromagnetic Energy

Frequency

Electromagnetic energy represents one mechanism by which prayer can be transformed into healing power. Although all humans generate such energy, spiritual healers seem to be unique (13). For example, whereas most people emit a variable electromagnetic frequency from their hands, healers emit a *steady* 7.8 Hz frequency (Hz, or hertz, is the number of waves that pass a fixed point per unit of time, i.e., cycles per second).

Perhaps because it is identical to the Earth's resonant frequency, this frequency appears to have special healing significance. For example, in mice it can heal cancer induced using a lower frequency. This indicates that some frequencies are life enhancing and others are not. Touch healers have been shown to transmit this 7.8 Hz, life-enhancing frequency to others through prayerlike consciousness.

Voltage

The body's cumulative electrical potential can be immense. Researchers have shown that spiritual healers' hands can emit more than 200 volts; nonhealers produced no more than 4 volts (13). Because such voltages are approximately 1 billion times stronger than brain-wave voltages and 100 million times stronger than those in the heart, their potential impact on the human body is enormous. It is conceivable for healers to "raise the dead" like defibrillators.

Human Energy Fields

Energy fields surround the human body (13, 14, 15). Most people at some level can sense them. It explains the intuitive feelings one has for another, including instant dislikes or physical chemistry. The halos surrounding spiritual beings in many traditions supposedly represent one higher manifestation of these fields. Barbara Brennan, a former NASA physicist, has developed a training program to enhance people's inherent capability to perceive these fields (14). A classic demonstration of these energy fields is called the "phantom leaf effect." After a part of a leaf has been cut off and destroyed, a precise image of the entire leaf can be obtained using Kirlian photography.

Proponents believe that the human energy field is composed of consecutive layers representing increasing energy vibration (Figure 9-1). Intersecting the body and the energy field are seven tornado-like energy centers called chakras. Fundamental to many Eastern healing traditions, these chakras bring in energy from the universal energy field and transform it into energy that the body can use. Located in front of the spinal cord, a power column or pranic tube receives life-force energy from the chakras and transmits it vertically through the body. Any energy imbalance or blockage eventually causes illness (basically, the theory behind acupuncture). Energy imbalances can be measured and assessed before the onset of physical disease by a number of devices.

Energy Fields and SCI

According to Sherry Pae, a teacher at the Barbara Brennan School of Healing, spinal cord injury will greatly affect energy flow through the body because of the cord's proximity to the power column. Furthermore, after injury the energy received by the base and sacral chakras is substantially reduced. The effects of the injury are stored in the *etheric field*, the energy field closest to the body. This field contains the template or blueprint for the physical body, duplicating every body cell and organ. As such, it is responsible for the growth, development, and repair of the physical body. If the etheric template is distorted, its physical product, the body, will also be distorted in some sense. After injury, the etheric field's dysfunctional energy vectors must be mended to facilitate physiological healing. Because

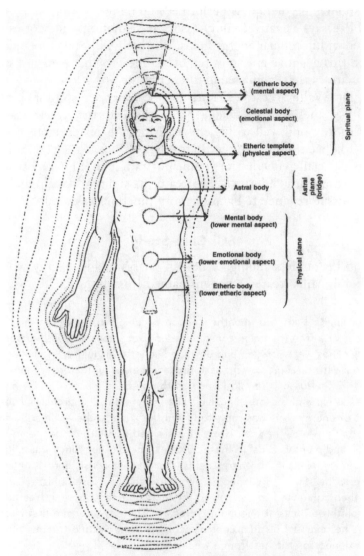

Figure 9-1 The human energy field is composed of consecutive layers representing increasing energy vibration. (From *Hands of Light* by Barbara Brennan, illustrated by Jos. A. Smith, Bantam Books. Used with permission.)

time tends to lock in a spinal cord injury within the etheric field, the sooner the therapy is performed the better.

Pae says negative, injury-associated emotional memories are stored within cellular energy fields. The body will heal more quickly when this negative energy is removed. She says that pain and spasticity are especially amenable to energy therapy.

Dr. Walter Weston is a prayer researcher and spiritual healer, who uses these energy fields (13). He believes that recent trauma injuries respond well to his efforts. Although his experience with SCI has been limited, he indicates that his healing therapies have been especially effective for traumatic brain injury. He reports that many severe head injuries he has treated have survived with damaged brain tissue regenerated and memory functions restored.

SCI Case Study

Using her understanding of human energy fields, energy worker Deborah Mills treated a patient named Russell:

According to Mills, four months after he became a paraplegic when he fell out of a tree (personal communication, December 9, 1998), Russell's energy lines were "broken and unwound" due to his injury. Her initial efforts were directed toward restoring and balancing the energy movement within Russell's physical body. With one hand placed on his pelvis near the hip and the other near his knee, she created a circular movement of energy. This was repeated from the knee to the ankle and again from the ankle to the foot. Next, Mills treated Russell's etheric, emotional, and mental fields. In these sessions, she did not touch Russell but placed her hands in his energy fields. In a manner consistent with many healers, she stated, "I connected my higher self to Russell's higher self and then connected to the universal energy source." Deborah treated Russell three times at one-month intervals. The day after the first treatment, he regained bladder control; soon after the second treatment, he transitioned to crutches from a wheelchair.

Regeneration Potential

Various animal studies support the theory that energy fields possess the blueprint for the physical body. For example, salamanders are able to regenerate severed limbs, including the tail, which contains spinal-cord segments. After amputation, electrical voltages can be measured around the missing parts. If the voltage exceeds a certain threshold, as is often the case in younger animals, regeneration occurs. Children also appear to have this capability. Specifically, they can regenerate the severed tip of a finger, including the same fingerprint. Given these results, it is not inconceivable that the therapeutic manipulation of energy fields could enhance the regenerative potential of an injured spinal cord.

From the Heart?

Healers believe that strong emotions are stored in energy fields and that the heart has access to them through the heart chakra. Dr. Paul Pearsall observed that many heart transplant recipients assume the donor's uniquely idiosyncratic behaviors, including musical tastes, food preferences, sexual desires, and vocabulary usage (16). Pearsall speculates that in addition to the brain, all of the body's 75 trillion cells have some sort of memory ability. The heart's cellular memory potential is especially significant because it is the body's most powerful energy generator, and its millions of cells beat in unison. Pearsall cites experiments showing a simultaneous synchronization and exchange of heart energy between noninteracting individuals sitting in the same room. Consistent with the heart's poetic role, this energy resonates between individuals like tuning forks.

This ability to exchange information with others, combined with the heart's ability to remember, provides one possible explanation on how prayer may influence another person. Investigations by Jack Stucki, a biofeedback and prayer researcher discussed in Part 1, further underscore the heart's potential importance. His studies suggest that prayer, even at great distance, can modify the electrical activity on the body where the heart chakra is located.

Collective Consciousness

Paul Pearsall speculates that the synchronization of heart energy between individuals provides one mechanism for obtaining group or collective consciousness. He refers to an often-quoted example of collective consciousness called the "100-monkey syndrome." In this example, on islands off Japan, one monkey learned a new skill. In turn, this monkey taught this skill to other monkeys. After the critical mass of 100 monkeys had been taught, suddenly all of them knew the skill, even those on nearby islands with no physical contact. Experiments have documented this effect in humans.

Experts theorize that collective consciousness is catalytic and self-feeding. As such, experts believe that if the collective consciousness represents a negative emotion, it adversely affects society. For example, in a strengthen-what-you-oppose perspective, a flu epidemic would be aggravated by the fear-based collective consciousness associated with catching the virus. Perhaps an understanding of collective consciousness can help explain why two million people who enter a hospital each year acquire infections they did not have when they went there. Does an infectious consciousness exist in addition to the disease?

On the other hand, if a group consciousness represents positive emotions like love, empathy, and compassion, it is humanity enhancing. Einstein showed that mass is just another form of energy. Consciousness, itself, is energy. It follows then that consciousness can create our physical reality, especially when collectively amplified.

When reflected in prayer, group consciousness can facilitate powerful healing. British physicist and theologian Dr. John Polkinghorne compares group prayer to laser light, which is powerful because its waves are in synchrony. As discussed by Walter Weston, synchronizing energy fields can generate immense, exponential power (13). For example, the power of two people praying would be four times that of a single person (2 × 2), and the power of 10 people praying would be 100 times that of a single person (10 × 10). A large church congregation of 1,000 unified in prayer would have 1 million times the praying power of a single person (1,000 × 1,000). Given the potential healing provided through group prayer, mechanisms have been established in which people can be prayed for by groups (17).

Conclusions

Modern medicine historically has viewed the human body as a collection of parts that must function, and as a result must be healed like a machine. Within this view of health, spirituality has no role. In contrast, spirituality is an integral part of many holistic, alternative healing traditions. Perhaps this is one reason why so many Americans have been turning to these traditions. They want to be treated from a mind–body–spirit perspective—and are listening to their hearts.

Additional Readings and Resources

In addition to the resources listed in Part 1, see the following:

Books

Brennan BA. *Hands of Light: A Guide to Healing Through the Human Energy Field.* New York: Bantam Books, 1988.

Hunt VV. *Infinite Mind: Science of the Human Vibrations of Consciousness.* Malibu, Calif.: Mailbu Publishing, 1996.

Pearsall P. *The Heart's Code: The New Findings about Cellular Memories and Their Role in the Mind/Body/Spirit Connection.* New York: Broadway Books, 1998.

Pert CB. *Molecules of Emotion: The Science Behind Mind-Body Medicine.* New York: Simon and Schuster, 1997.

Weston W. *How Prayer Heals.* Charlottesville, Va.: Hampton Roads Publishing, 1998.

MIND INSTRUCTION:
CONSCIOUSNESS-BASED HEALING

The Mind-Instructor Clinic in London, England, treats a variety of neurological disorders including spinal cord injury and dysfunction. Developed by clinic director Hratch Ogali, the program's underlying philosophy of consciousness-driven healing is difficult to explain with conventional, body-focused, biomedical concepts and must be described more through the mind–body–spirit healing wisdom inherent in many of the world's older healing traditions.

Introduction

Hratch Ogali stresses rigorous strengthening exercises—just as other rehabilitation programs do that are emerging for SCI. However, the program's foundation is based on a shift in patient consciousness, catalyzed and reinforced by Ogali, from the defeating "you-will-never-walk-again" and other negative, recovery-inhibiting attitudes that are deeply imprinted in consciousness after injury to a positive "Yeah, I *will* do it." When this new attitude is embedded with conviction in our consciousness—the captain of our ship—the physical body starts to follow. Ogali's role is catalytic; he is not the healer but metaphorically the force that opens the prison door

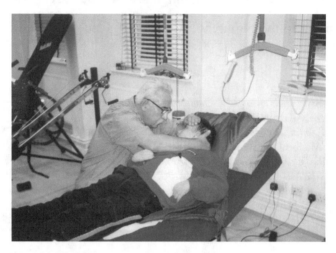

Figure 9-2   Hratch Ogali treats a patient at his Mind Instructor Clinic in London, England. (Photo taken by Laurance Johnston.)

allowing the patient to step through if so desired. It is the patient who heals himself or herself, starting from the deepest soul level.

Demonstrating the neuronal adaptability (i.e., plasticity) that scientists now believe is inherent in all, Ogali speculates that nascent neuronal growth commences, dormant neurons turn on, and new neuronal connections are created. Regardless of the specific intervening physiological mechanisms, Ogali believes that physical healing stems from the healing in consciousness, which is then reinforced through aggressive physical rehabilitation (Figure 9-2). According to Ogali, most patients who have persevered with his demanding program have accrued additional function—sometimes subtle but life-enhancing, and sometimes dramatic.

Over the past year, Ogali's program has received extensive press attention in the United Kingdom (18), and also was the focus of a Discovery Health Channel documentary called *Miracle Steps* featuring Christopher Reeve (19). Much of this media attention has revolved around Gemma, a 19-year-old woman who sustained a complete cervical C2-3 injury in an auto accident when she was 7. After treatment by Ogali, Gemma can now initiate movement with effort in much of her body below the injury site for the first time since injury, including standing and taking up to 20 steps. As would be expected for such an unconventional, consciousness-directed program, the British SCI biomedical establishment has been skeptical and dismissed Gemma's progress as a development that might have occurred anyway. In *Miracles Steps*, Gemma succinctly responds: "Medicine didn't make me take a step; this guy did." (19)

Given my mission to explore therapies that expand the SCI-healing spectrum, Ogali invited me to visit his clinic and observe first hand his approach. Over four days, I watched him treat people with SCI and a diversity of other neurological disorders, including ALS (Lou Gehrig's disease), traumatic brain injury (TBI), and rare developmental disorders in children, such as adrenoleukodystrophy (ALD), a myelin disorder featured in the movie *Lorenzo's Oil*. Ogali has treated more than 50 individuals with SCI, as well as many with multiple sclerosis (MS).

Hratch Ogali

Age 55, Hratch Ogali is of Armenian descent and grew up in the Middle East before immigrating to England as a young man. As a severe dyslexic, he finds in-depth reading challenging. Demonstrating once again that many disabilities are the source of strength, Ogali's perceptions on disability come from a different view of the universe than conventionally trained doctors and scientists, who acquire much of their knowledge through reading text books and journals. Denied traditional sources of knowledge, Ogali's intuitive insights that evolved into his program came from 14 years of extensive contemplative meditation. Although Western science eschews such a process for acquiring knowledge, ancient-based cultures embrace it as the only effective way for obtaining higher-level insight (e.g., Native-American vision quests, Indian yogic experiences, early Christian mystics, etc).

Perhaps reflecting the inner peace that accrues from such cumulative meditation, Ogali has a gentle, almost sagelike attitude when interacting with his patients. He treats them with love and develops a seemingly soul intimacy that creates the connection needed to generate healing in consciousness. Ogali's clinic is located in the heart of London several blocks from Sherlock Holmes' Baker Street and a mile from Buckingham Palace. In a setting conducive for fostering spirit-driven healing, the clinic is housed in a former presbytery for the attached St. James' Cathedral.

Psychoneuroimmunology

As a biochemist who was for many years a senior official at the National Institutes of Health (NIH), I once embraced, like most of my colleagues, a mechanistic model of healing that essentially viewed the body as a summation of parts, whether they are molecules, cells, or organs. Under such a model, consciousness has no role.

Although the scientific community traditionally disdains mind–body–spirit healing, it has grudgingly acknowledged a more scientific-sounding discipline (a rose by any other name) called psychoneuroimmunology, which to some degree conceptually represents the same thing—that is, how attributes of consciousness, such as emotions, attitudes, and so forth, affect health. Ogali himself states that it is difficult to describe what he does: "There is no description that you can give to what takes place; it will always seem mystical and mysterious. Yet to me, it is a simple calculation of the mind and the brain working under instruction to create change." (19)

The Role of Consciousness

The role of consciousness or the mind in healing always has been troublesome for scientists. The 17th century French philosopher René Descartes framed the contemporary debate on the subject by stating that everything under the sun consists of either *res cognitas* (i.e., consciousness, mind) or *res extensa* (i.e., physical matter) (20).

Unlike neuroscientists who tend to equate consciousness with brain chemistry and biology, many alternative healing traditions view the brain more from Descartes' perspective; specifically, the brain is merely the body's physical processor for consciousness. Within this view, although possessing a good processor affects your overt intelligence and although outward expression of consciousness may be a function of processor's neuronal synaptic connections, and so forth, it is not the site of your consciousness anymore than your big toe is. With such beliefs, even if our brain is damaged from severe head injury, stroke, ALS, MS, or Alzheimer's disease, our consciousness is always whole and complete; and, relevant to Ogali's work, it possesses the blueprint memories of our able-bodied selves that can be accessed for healing.

However, all the disability-related negative attitudes and emotions that may have been picked up interfere with accessing these healing blueprints. Like burrs sticking to Velcro, these beliefs are difficult to eliminate and, unfortunately, often are imposed by our medical professionals. Professionally, it is called crepe-hanging, as at a funeral. For example, when a cancer patient is told he has only six months to live, indeed he often dies after that time period because that expectation has been imprinted in his consciousness by an authority figure.

For SCI, the imprint is even deeper because it is based on medicine's cumulative historical experience for the disorder and not the ever-growing possibilities of the future. Patients are told they will never walk again and any thoughts otherwise will just prevent them from getting on with their lives. That is a tough, deeply imprinted sentence that must be surmounted in order to have significant physical healing. It is like trying to push a car in one direction (i.e., healing the physical body) when the steering wheel (i.e., your consciousness) is cranked in another direction. Any healing modality will work better when the steering wheel is turned in the right direction—basically, Ogali's goal.

According to Gemma, in addition to busting apart the pervasive you-will-never-walk-again attitude, Ogali made her "deal with a lot of painful memories and remember how it was to move." As Gemma watched her siblings and friends move on with their lives, her resentment and dislike of herself grew; she notes, however, Ogali "made me like myself again." (19)

In *Miracle Steps*, Ogali summarized his approach:

> I basically teach natural wisdom: how the mind, body and spirit work together; what kind of power we possess; what kind of creativity we possess; how we can use that creativity to activate, bring to life, to create something new. And when the mind becomes free, the mind is capable.

He adds, "The mind is all spirit. Spirit remembers everything, including how it built the body; it knows." (19)

Mind Instruction

One key program element is a guided meditation session. Because the session's purpose is to establish a one-on-one communion of consciousness between Ogali and patient, I did not observe them; however, I had my own session. Although I have meditated for years, I have rarely gone into a deeper, trancelike state. It is in such a receptive state that Ogali begins the process of busting apart the negative belief patterns that inhibit physical healing. To help further germinate these nascent seeds of consciousness, such sessions are periodically held. Reinforcing these private sessions, Ogali continues his mind instructions in the more routine physical-therapy sessions. Gemma's father, Mike, felt like an intruder when present, because such a bond had been created between his daughter and Ogali (19). I often felt the same way in my observations.

Furthermore, Ogali's soothing mind instructions frequently spilled over into my consciousness. As he encouraged patients to relax their muscles, I was soon nodding off. This reaction became ridiculous when I nearly dropped my coffee after Ogali gently instructed Alan, a C-2 injury, to relax his severely contracted left shoulder. I was told that Ogali's soporific influence on observers was common. Given such a bystander effect, I suspect its effect on the patient who is the actual target of the instructions is substantial.

These mind instructions, however, are of relatively limited value unless the patient carries out extensive daily reinforcement of breathing, meditative, and mental-concentration exercises, which are individually tailored to help replace the old thinking with the new healing paradigm in the patient's consciousness. Although uniquely developed by Ogali, meditative breathing exercises are, in fact, a key component of many Eastern healing practices, such as qigong and scalp acupuncture as discussed in chapter 2 of this book.

Energy Work

In addition to his consciousness-influencing efforts, Ogali views himself as a hands-on energy worker, a concept also discussed in the preceding section. He believes we are all fundamentally electromagnetic beings who are a part of, or connected to, a greater electromagnetic universe; this electromagnetic relationship can be used for healing.

Ogali claims to tap into our ubiquitous electromagnetic universe and then "activates the brain . . . by penetrating the magnetic energy of patients, who instantly feel some sort of sensations in their legs and feet." This gives Ogali a sense of the patient's residual function, which he then exploits and builds upon through further energy and physical therapy. Ogali states: "If you have one-percent function, you can have two percent" and so on.

Physical Therapy

Although Ogali's mind instruction is carried out on an ongoing basis, much of his program involves intense physical exercise and conditioning. At this point, Ogali's once empathetic manner turns into that of a bust-your-behind motivational coach. Although his clinic contains a variety of standard strengthening and rehabilitation equipment, Ogali emphasizes conditioning on a semirecumbent hand and leg cycle and the use of a body-supporting hoist for walking efforts. Ogali believes that SCI-associated spasms should not be suppressed but exploited to stimulate functional recovery. With this belief, patients are encouraged to gradually wean themselves from spasticity-controlling medications, which Ogali views as reducing the body's sensitivity to the mind's healing instructions.

Overall, this program requires a substantial commitment effort. In addition to carrying out time-consuming mind-instructor exercises that require discipline, the program requires considerable physical work. Although Gemma's functional recovery was dramatic given her injuries, it required many months of dedicated, focused work that pushed other activities to the background.

Physiological Explanations

In spite of the program's radical nature, scientific findings to some degree are consistent with Ogali's patients' functional recovery. First, neurophysiological assessments show that most clinically classified complete injuries have some intact, albeit perhaps dormant, neurons running through the injury site. Second, studies indicate that you need only a small percentage of working neurons to have fairly substantial function. Third, the spinal cord and interacting neuronal networks are physiologically much more complex than originally thought, suggesting the function-stimulating integration of different neuronal systems above and below the injury site. Finally, a number of aggressive rehabilitation programs have triggered some restored function in individuals with chronic SCI, including the late Christopher Reeve. All these findings suggest possibilities of how

Ogali's program, which taps into the patient's will at the deepest level, restores some function

Conclusions

Although it is difficult to explain from a conventional biomedical context, the Mind-Instructor program reflects healing wisdom embraced by mankind through most of history until the emergence of modern medicine. Even if modern medicine acknowledges the role of consciousness through disciplines such as psychoneuroimmunology, it is ill equipped to assess the healing potential. Specifically, medicine's most powerful analytical tool—the randomized double-blind clinical trial—is worthless for measuring consciousness' healing effects. For example, what would be a standardized dose of consciousness and what would be the placebo? Hence, consciousness, perhaps the most powerful component in our healing armamentarium, is off the radar screen when it comes to science's preferred way of looking at the world.

Most of us, however, intuitively understand that our consciousness, our will, and our mental and emotional attitudes affect the outcome of whatever we strive for, ranging from athletic performance to rehabilitation. Given such understanding, little of Ogali's mind-influencing, soul-motivating, function-restoring program is truly radical.

Additional Readings and Resources

Books

Pert CB. *Molecules of Emotion: The Science behind Mind-Body Medicine.* New York: Simon and Schuster, 1997.

Internet

Mind-Instructor Clinic: www.mindinstructor.com

Videos

Miracle Steps produced by and available through Advanced Medical Productions, 307 W. Weaver St., Carrboro, NC 27510 (www.advancedmedical.tv)

REFERENCES

1. Dossey L. *Prayer is Good Medicine*. New York: HarperCollins, 1996.
2. Marwick C. Should physicians prescribe prayer for health? *JAMA* 1995; 273: 1561–1562.
3. Koenig HG. *Is Religion Good for Your Health?* Binghamton: Haworth Press, 1997.
4. Benor DJ. Survey of spiritual healing research. *Complementary Medical Research* 1990; 4(3): 9–33.
5. Dossey L. *Healing Words: The Power of Prayer and the Practice of Medicine*. New York: HarperCollins, 1993.
6. Braden G. *Walking Between the Worlds: the Science of Compassion*. Bellevue, Wa.: Radio Bookstore Press, 1997.
7. Lipton B. Insight into cellular consciousness. *Bridges* 2001; 12(1): 1, 4–6.
8. Byrd RC. Positive therapeutic effects of intercessory prayer in a coronary care unit population. *Southern Medical Journal* 1988; 81: 826–829.
9. Harris WS, Gowada M, Kolb JW, et al. A randomized, controlled trial of the effects of remote, intercessory prayer on outcomes in patients admitted to the coronary care unity. *Arch Intern Med* 1999; 159: 2273–2278.
10. Targ E. Distant healing. *IONS Noetic Sciences Review* 1999; 49: 24–39.
11. Benor DJ. *Healing Research: Holistic Energy Medicine and Spirituality Vol. 1*. Deddington, Oxfordshire, UK: Helix 1993.
12. Weston W. *How Prayer Heals*. Charlottesville, Va: Hampton Roads Publishing, 1998.
13. Weston W. *How Prayer Heals*. Charlottesville, Va.: Hampton Roads Publishing, 1998.
14. Brennan BA. *Hands of Light: A Guide to Healing Through the Human Energy Field*. New York: Bantam Books, 1988.
15. Hunt VV. *Infinite Mind: Science of the Human Vibrations of Consciousness*. Malibu, Calif.: Malibu Publishing, 1996.
16. Pearsall, P. *The Heart's Code: The New Findings about Cellular Memories and Their Role in the Mind/Body/Spirit Connection*. New York: Broadway Books, 1998.
17. Dossey L. *Prayer Is Good Medicine*. New York: HarperCollins, 1996.
18. Mind-Instructor Clinic. Available online at www.mindinstructor.com
19. *Miracle Steps* Carrboro, NC: Advanced Medical Productions, 2004.
20. Koch C. Thinking about the conscious mind. *Science* 2004; 306: 979–980.

10

SCI Health Problems

NATURAL URINARY TRACT HEALTH

This chapter discusses various natural alternatives that fight urinary-tract infections (UTIs), and, by so doing, help preserve the future effectiveness of life-saving antibiotics.

UTIs can be an aggravating, recurring health problem for individuals with spinal cord injury (SCI). According to the Agency for Health Care Policy and Research, 80% of those with SCI will experience UTIs within 16 years of injury; UTIs are the most frequent secondary medical complication during acute care and rehabilitation: and urinary-system disorders are the fifth most common primary or secondary cause of death (1). In the general population, about 90% of UTIs are caused by *E. coli* bacteria, which although a normal part of our intestinal miroflora, do not belong in our urinary system. In the case of SCI, other bacteria in addition to *E. coli* can cause UTIs (2).

Antibiotics: Double-Edged Sword?

For more than half a century, people with SCI have relied on antibiotics to control UTIs. The development of antibiotics stems back to 1928 when British microbiologist and eventual Nobel laureate Alexander Fleming observed that bacterial growth was inhibited by a mold that was later shown to produce penicillin. Although infection-fighting molds have been a part of humankind's healing armamentarium since antiquity and noted by scientists before Fleming, penicillin became the first antibiotic isolated from one. The exigencies of World War II resulted in penicillin's production in sufficient quantities for general use. Since then, scientists have developed a multitude of potent antibiotics. In my case, as a graduate student, I help elucidate the molecular mechanism of vancomycin (3), now an antibiotic of last resort in resistant infections.

Although antibiotics have greatly increased the life expectancy of people with SCI, reliance on them has ominous future implications given the growth of antibiotic-resistant bacteria. For example, every year, two million hospital patients acquire infections that they did not have when they entered the hospital; of these, 80,000 die (4). Statistics such as these are especially relevant to infection- and hospitalization-prone individuals with SCI and clearly indicate the need to maintain antibiotic effectiveness.

In spite of their clear importance, every time we use antibiotics we short-circuit our body's inherent healing potential, cumulatively compromising our long-term health. We may be winning the immediate health-care battle, but we are setting ourselves up to lose the war. Furthermore, in spite of commonly held assumptions that bacteria are the "bad guys," optimal health requires that we maintain a symbiotic, health-enhancing partnership with them. For example, many different bacteria that live within our digestive system are essential for proper digestion and chronic health. Every time we use an antibiotic, we undercut this bacterial partnership. By killing off the good guys, we create a void that may be filled by health-compromising pathogens or antibiotic-resistant bacteria that now have no competition for growth.

Emphasizing this theme, a 2003 *Science* magazine article stated: "Not only does the highly evolved gut flora community extend the processing of undigested food to the benefit of the host, but it also contributes to host defense by limiting colonization of the gastrointestinal tract by pathogens." (5) The article notes that at least 500 different microbes live in our gut.

Unfortunately, we also face tremendous exposure to antibiotic residues through meat and poultry consumption. In this country annually, 25 million pounds of antibiotics (eight times human medical use) are fed to livestock and poultry, not for therapeutic reasons but to promote economic-efficient growth. By fostering development of resistant bacteria, this practice may ultimately render useless the antibiotics that have been a cornerstone of SCI health care. The World Health Organization has recommended that this procedure be discontinued, and reflecting this recommendation, the European Union has ordered its member countries to end the practice by 2006 (6).

To reduce your vulnerability to the seemingly inevitable erosion of antibiotic power, use when feasible and prudent various alternatives for enhancing urinary-tract health and attempt to hold in reserve the heavy-duty antibiotic artillery for major medical crises. For most of these innocuous alternatives, there is little to lose and potentially much to gain.

Nutritional Approaches

Cranberries and Blueberries

Cranberry products are a traditional UTI-fighting folk remedy that has been embraced by the SCI community. In addition to acidifying urine, cranberries contain substances that inhibit bacteria from attaching to the bladder lining, promoting the flushing out of bacteria with the urine stream. These antibacterial substances include tanninlike compounds called proanthocyanidins and the sugar D-mannose (see the text that follows).

Cranberries' UTI-fighting ability is supported by an ever-growing body of scientific evidence. Although more research is needed on SCI-associated UTIs, a pilot study indicated that drinking cranberry juice greatly reduced bacterial attachment to cells lining the bladder in subjects with SCI (7). Promisingly, this was a broad-spectrum, antibacterial effect not limited merely to *E. coli*, the culprit of most UTIs in the general population.

To avoid excess sugar consumption, consume unsweetened—albeit lip-puckering—cranberry juice, cranberry-extract capsules, or naturally sweet blueberries, which contain similar UTI-fighting substances.

D-Mannose

Studies suggest that D-mannose is even more effective than cranberries in dislodging *E. coli* bacteria from the bladder wall (8, 9, 10, 11), supposedly ameliorating more than 90% of UTIs in 24 to 48 hours. In addition to reading many impressive testimonials from able-bodied consumers whose recurring UTI's have been successfully treated with the product, I talked to several D-mannose users with SCI: Stephanie, an artist with paraplegia who has had recurring UTIs, says D-mannose was "a wonderful UTI product." She adds "I take several glasses of water a day with a half teaspoon of the powdered D-mannose. I am absolutely positive that it has stabilized my bladder condition to the effect of better control, easier to empty, and the discomfort 'tightness' or burning is gone."

Richard, a retired teacher, told me that his UTI frequency had greatly increased with age until he was afflicted routinely with one that required antibiotic therapy every 40 days. About a year ago, he started taking D-mannose prophylactically and feels it has made a huge difference, noting that "most of the time now, my urine is more clear and lacking of the characteristic UTI-associated odor." He says the product has greatly decreased his UTI incidence. David, a Washington, DC administrative official, stated that he is a "D-mannose fan." He notes "I've had numerous urinary tract infections for 25 years and was starting to run out of effective antibiotics. Since I started taking it six months ago, I've not had a UTI."

D-mannose is a naturally occurring sugar similar in structure to, but metabolized differently from, glucose (a component of table sugar). Because the body metabolizes only small amounts of D-mannose and excretes the rest in the urine, it doesn't interfere with blood-sugar regulation, even in diabetics. The cell wall of the *E. coli* bacteria has tiny fingerlike projections that contain complex molecules called lectins on their surfaces. These lectins are cellular glue that binds the bacteria to the bladder wall so they cannot be rinsed out readily by urination. However, because D-mannose molecules will glom on to these lectins and fill up all of the bacterial anchoring sites, the bacteria can no longer attach to the bladder wall and are flushed away. In other words, unlike antibiotics, D-mannose does not kill any bacteria, whether they are good or bad, but simply helps to displace them. Visualize the bacteria as burrs sticking to the lining of your clothes unless the clothes are so covered with lint that the burrs fall away. Essentially, D-mannose represents the molecular lint that makes the bacterial burrs fall away from your urinary-tract lining.

Herbal Medicine

Before modern medicine started emphasizing chemically synthe-sized drugs, herbal remedies were the cornerstone of most of the world's healing traditions. Even today, herbal remedies are used by 80% of the world's population who cannot afford Western pharma-ceuticals (Figure 10-1). As concern grows about adverse drug side effects, more than one third of all Americans are once again turning to herbal remedies to treat diverse ailments, including UTIs (12).

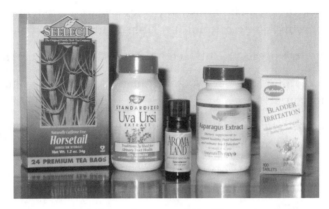

Figure 10-1 Many herbal remedies treat UTIs. (Photo taken by Laurance Johnston.)

Many urinary-system herbal remedies have a long history of use by both Western and indigenous (e.g., Native American) cultures; have been listed in numerous official medical resources before our focus on synthesized drugs pushed them to the sidelines; and even today, often have been sanctioned by European governments in efforts to reconcile and integrate herbal and modern medicine perspectives. Although little focus has been on the use of these herbal remedies to treat SCI-specific UTIs, many of these remedies act against *E. coli* bacteria, the primary UTI culprit in the general and SCI population. Available as capsules, extracts, tinctures, herbal infusions and teas, or combination products, several UTI-fighting herbal remedies or medicinal foods are listed:

- *Uva Ursi* or bearberry, isolated from a small shrub related to blueberry and cranberry plants, contains a urinary antiseptic called arbutin.

- *Horsetail*, isolated from a prehistoric-looking plant that resembles a horse's tail, supports general urinary tract health.

- *Juniper berries* contain volatile oils that serve as urinary antiseptics.

- *Buchu*, an indigenous South African remedy often combined with cranberries in commercial products, contains volatile oils that are urinary-tract antiseptics.

- *Asparagus*, especially the wild type, is a traditional remedy for promoting urinary-tract health.

- *Parsley*, the familiar garnish, provides urinary-system nutritional support and contains apiol, a volatile oil urinary-tract antiseptic.

- *Celery seed* possesses antibacterial agents, including apiol.

- *Garlic*, an herbal heavyweight in many respects, has significant antibacterial activity.

- *Goldenseal root*, isolated from a North American woodland plant, contains an antibacterial compound called berberine.

- *Marshmallow root*, isolated from a plant that grows in wet, marshy areas, possesses a high mucilage content that soothes mucus membranes.

- *Corn silk*, prepared from the stigmas of corn plant female flowers, is valued for urinary system support.

- *Birch*, the deciduous tree, possesses many antibacterial substances.

- *Cleavers* (also called goosegrass), a common succulent plant, is beneficial for treating diverse urinary-system problems.

- *Hydrangea root*, isolated from the elegant shrub, contains substances that nutritionally support the urinary system.

Essential Oils

Often the antibacterial agents in herbs, volatile essential oils are extracted from plants using steam distillation and used in aromatherapy. These highly concentrated oils are complex mixtures of chemicals possessing wide-ranging properties. The chemicals in one drop of essential oil can be the equivalent to thirty cups of an herbal tea. Essential oils can fight diverse infections (13), including the *E. coli* bacteria. UTIs can be treated with baths and massages using, for example, sandalwood, pine, chamomile, cedarwood, juniper, bergamot, fennel oils, tea tree, niaouli, and cajeput. For example, a massage oil containing sandalwood, niaouli, or cajeput can be rubbed directly over your lower abdomen above your pubic bone and lower back kidney region. These concentrated essential oils are usually diluted with some sort of vegetable oil or lotion before being applied to the skin.

Homeopathy

Although many homeopathic remedies are often confused with herbal products that bear similar names, these remedies are based on fundamentally different principles. Specifically, prepared by a process of a successive cycle of dilution and shaking, homeopathic remedies (unlike herbal or essential oil remedies) are virtually bereft of physiologically active molecules. Homeopathy's healing effects are mediated through a retained energy imprint of the original, predilution substance.

Ideally, in order to obtain the most effective remedies, see a professional homeopath (14), who will attempt to assign remedies based on your unique symptoms. However, if this is not feasible, many homeopathic remedies are indicated for UTIs, including Aconitum napellus, Apis, Berberis, Belladonna, Cantharis, Equisetum, Eupatorium purpureum, Mercurius vivus, Nitric acid, Nux vomica, Pulsatilla, and Sarsaparilla. In order to make the decision easier, many readily available urinary-tract homeopathic products have combined a number of these individual remedies.

Conclusions

To help preserve the future effectiveness of life-saving antibiotics, consider using when prudent natural alternatives to enhance urinary-tract health, such as cranberries, blueberries, D-mannose, and herbal, homeopathic, and essential-oil remedies. Who knows? You may lose your "UTI chill on blueberry fill."

Resources

All of the UTI-fighting alternatives discussed in this chapter can be obtained from nutritional stores or Internet sources.

NATURAL PROSTATE HEALTH

Spinal cord injury predominately affects men. Although society tends to focus on the loss of ambulation as the foremost SCI concern, when asked about their priorities, men consistently indicate that SCI-associated sexual and reproductive dysfunction is just as important. As such, the last thing that a male with SCI needs is to have his compromised function further aggravated by prostate disorders.

Affecting not just elderly men, prostate disorders are much more common than would be expected in middle-aged individuals. For example, over half of men ages 40 to 59 have enlarged prostates, and although most will not develop clinically significant disease, one fourth of 50-year-olds have some cancerous cells in their prostate. This chapter will highlight various prostate-enhancing nutritional, herbal, or alternative approaches that may help one avert more serious pharmaceutical and surgical therapies.

The prostate, located below the bladder, is a walnut-size gland that produces seminal fluid. Because the gland surrounds the urethra that drains the bladder, prostate disorders often affect urination. The three most common disorders are (a) an inflammatory infection called prostatitis; (b) benign prostatic hyperplasia (BPH), a prevalent noncancerous enlargement of the prostate; and (c) cancer, the most frequent male malignancy. Prostate disorders are associated with age-related changes in steroid sex hormones. After age 40, testosterone declines, and a testosterone variant called dihydrotestosterone (DHT) and the female-associated hormone estrogen increase. DHT stimulates cell growth and in turn, prostate enlargement. By inhibiting DHT elimination, estrogen has the same effect.

Food and Nutrient Supplements

Prostate dysfunction has been called a nutritional disease. It is much more common in developed Western countries that emphasize cooked meats, pasteurized dairy products, and eggs, all foods that tend to accumulate environmental toxins. In contrast, fruit- and vegetable-rich diets exert a protective effect.

Scientific studies are challenging some entrenched views on what we have traditionally considered nutritionally wholesome foods. For example, evidence suggests that pasteurized milk may be bad for the prostate. Overall, countries that consume the most pasteurized milk have the highest incidence of prostate cancer (15). The culprit may be milk's calcium. Excessive calcium intake, regardless of source, apparently suppresses the synthesis of a form of vitamin D that inhibits prostate cancer.

In contrast, men who consume tomatoes, tomato-based foods (e.g., ketchup, pasta with spaghetti sauce, etc.), guavas, watermelon, and pink grapefruit are less likely to get prostate cancer. These foods contain a powerful antioxidant, prostate-enhancing agent called *lycopene* (16) that gives them their characteristic red color. Available as a nutritional supplement, lycopene not only prevents prostate cancer but also may reduce existing tumor size. Another prostate-protecting food is fructose, the sugar in fruit that is used to sweeten many foods. Overall, its consumption is associated with a reduced prostate-cancer risk. Unlike calcium, fructose stimulates the production of a form of vitamin D that inhibits tumors (17).

Several trace nutrients that are often deficient in our diet also enhance prostate health. For example, a lack of zinc especially affects the prostate because this gland uses it much more than any other body part. By altering steroid hormone metabolism, zinc supplementation can reduce prostate enlargement. Interestingly, pumpkin seeds, a traditional folk remedy for promoting male reproductive and prostate health, are rich in zinc. Selenium is another often-deficient trace nutrient that is essential for prostate health (18). Increasing selenium intake, whether through supplements or selenium-rich foods (e.g., Brazil nuts), has been shown to reduce prostate-cancer risk.

Other foods or nutritional factors that inhibit prostate cancer include vitamin D (19); vitamin E, an antioxidant that inhibits cancer growth (20); garlic, onions, and scallions, which possess cancer-fighting, sulfur-containing compounds (21); and red wine, which contains the cancer-fighting agent resveratol (22).

Herbal Remedies

In Europe, herbal remedies are widely used to treat prostate disorders. In America, however, a regulatory charade makes these remedies available by pretending that they are merely dietary supplements. Because of the extensive scientific base that often supports their use, they are much more than folk remedies.

Foremost among these herbs is saw palmetto, isolated from the berries of a small palm tree common to the U.S.'s southeastern coastal region. A traditional Native-American remedy, saw palmetto reduces prostate enlargement by inhibiting the synthesis of growth-stimulating DHT and promoting DHT elimination by lowering estrogen levels. Many clinical studies demonstrate saw palmetto's effectiveness. In fact, the herb works better in treating prostate enlargement than the frequently prescribed drug Proscar. Specifically, saw palmetto was shown to be effective in nearly 90% of patients after 4 to 6 weeks, whereas Proscar works in fewer than half the patients after a year (23). And because the drug is less effective, much more expensive, and its major side effect is erectile dysfunction, choosing saw palmetto seems self-evident.

Often administered with saw palmetto, another herbal heavy-weight is pygeum. An indigenous African remedy obtained from tree bark, studies indicate that pygeum can treat BPH and prostatitis (23, 24). The herb also contains chemicals that inhibit DHT-associated prostate enlargement. A third herbal remedy is Cernilton, a popular European product prepared from the extract of mainly rye pollen. Numerous studies document Cernilton's ability to treat BPH and prostatitis (25, 26, 27). Finally, stinging nettle is a traditional herbal folk remedy for many ailments, including prostate disorders. Clinical studies indicate that the herb (marketed as Bazoton in Europe) also can relieve BPH symptoms (28).

Homeopathy

Homeopathy, a popular alternative healing tradition, offers several remedies for prostate disorders. For example, according to the *Consumer Guide to Homeopathy* (29), homeopathic remedies for prostate disorders include Chimaphilla umbellata, Pulsatilla, Clematis, Apis, Staphysagria, Selenium, Baryta carb, Kali bic, and Causticum.

Sunlight

Despite concern about skin damage, studies have shown that sun exposure enhances prostate health (30, 31, 32) apparently by stimulating vitamin D production. For example, one study showed that men who had the least cumulative, lifetime sun exposure were more likely to get prostate cancer at a younger age.

Conclusions

One way or another, economic factors pervasively influence our health. For example, the dairy industry relentlessly promotes pasteurized milk's benefits to adults in spite of much evidence to the contrary, and ketchup producers now portray the condiment as a health food. It is hard to know whom to listen to. Unfortunately, physicians listen mostly to profit-motivated drug companies when it concerns our medicines and have had little training in nutritional, herbal, or alternative healing approaches. Even though safer, less expensive, and more effective options are often available; a blue-ribbon federal health advisory committee concluded that far too many prostate surgeries are being performed (33); and everyone complains about soaring medical costs, American men still spend billions of dollars annually on surgical and pharmaceutical treatments that often carry serious side effects. Knowledge is power. If we don't want economic factors influencing our health, we need to reclaim more responsibility for it and further educate ourselves on healing options.

Resources

You can purchase most of the referenced supplements and products at nutritional stores or through Internet sources.

Additional Readings and Resources

Books

Redmon GL. *Managing and Preventing Prostate Disorders: The Natural Alternatives.* Hohm Press: Prescott, Ariz., 2000.

NUTRITIONAL AND BOTANICAL APPROACHES TO DIABETES

Diabetes incidence has skyrocketed in recent decades as a result of our dietary and lifestyle choices; that is, we are too fat, eat bad foods, and don't exercise enough. Unfortunately, because of extensive metabolic-, hormonal-, body-composition shifts that occur after spinal cord injury, people with SCI are especially prone to developing diabetes. This chapter discusses various nutritional or botanical approaches that reduce blood-sugar levels in diabetics.

Overview

Diabetes is characterized by the body's inability to use glucose properly, the body's metabolic energy currency. Under healthy conditions, the hormone insulin controls blood-glucose levels. Produced by the pancreas, insulin flows through the blood to various tissues where they bind to cell-surface receptors. This binding initiates a complex biochemical cascade that culminates in glucose uptake into cells to fuel metabolic processes. As blood-glucose levels decline due to cellular uptake, the pancreas shuts down insulin production to prevent hypoglycemia (low blood sugar) and the liver, the body's nutrient-processing organ, starts releasing glucose back into the blood.

Although distinctions are more blurred than once thought, in type-1 or juvenile diabetes, the pancreas produces inadequate insulin to promote glucose uptake into cells. In contrast, in type-2, or adult-onset diabetes, cells become less responsive to the insulin that is still produced.

Through not clearly defined physiological mechanisms, persistently high blood-glucose may eventually lead to complications such as kidney disease, neuropathy (nerve disease), and eye problems.

Diabetes and SCI

Dr. William Bauman and colleagues at the Bronx VA Medical Center have shown that SCI predisposes one to diabetes (34, 35). For example, their research indicates that (a) only 44% of veterans with SCI have normal glucose metabolism compared to 82% without SCI, and (b) higher-level injuries further predispose one to diabetes.

Nutrient Density and SCI

Before our sedentary modern age, humans had high caloric needs due to more intense manual labor. If 4,000 calories per day were needed to fuel such labor, one was much more likely to absorb trace nutrients compared to today's office worker who gains weight from 1,500 calories a day of nutrient-depleted, processed foods. This concept is especially relevant to SCI. For example, by comparing identical twins with and without SCI, Bauman has shown that caloric needs are greatly reduced after injury (36). Such a reduction automatically results in the uptake of fewer trace nutrients in a weight-maintaining diet.

Another factor compromising nutrient uptake is extensive antibiotic use, which is a life-saving cornerstone of SCI medicine. A 2003 *Science* magazine article (37) noted: "Not only does the highly evolved gut flora community extend the processing of undigested food to the benefit of the host, but it also contributes to host defense by limiting colonization of the gastrointestinal tract by pathogens." More simply stated, there are hundreds of bacterial species within our gut that are essential for proper digestion. Every time one uses an antibiotic, assistive bacteria are killed, in turn, lessening the uptake of nutrients already inherently compromised by SCI.

The gist of this discussion is people with SCI need to make every calorie count because the adverse ramifications of eating nutrient-depleted food will be greatly magnified for them. Furthermore, given these considerations, the effectiveness of supplementing your diet with various nutrients to reduce blood-glucose levels depends on how much of the nutrients you already absorb from your diet. If your diet already contains an abundance of a nutrient, a supplement isn't going to help, but if the nutrient is lacking, a supplement may provide significant benefit. Many of the foods, supplements, or botanical agents discussed below are supported by scientific studies, including in some cases rigorous double-blind clinical studies. These supplements are readily available from nutrition and health-food or ethnic grocery stores, or from Internet sources (Figure 10-2).

Mineral Supplements

Trace amounts of chromium are essential for proper carbohydrate metabolism. Depending on dietary intake, studies suggest that chromium supplementation lowers blood-glucose levels by increasing cell-surface insulin receptors, and in turn glucose transport into

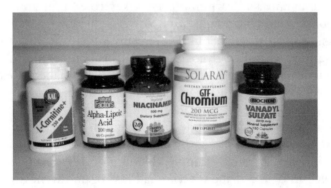

Figure 10-2 Various nutritional supplements have been shown to lower blood-sugar levels in diabetics. (Photo taken by Laurance Johnston.)

cells (38). Traditional food sources of chromium include beer, brewer's yeast, brown rice, cheese, meat, and whole grains.

Before insulin, vanadium was a traditional French diabetes remedy. Animal and human studies indicate that vanadium, like chromium, facilitates glucose uptake and metabolism by enhancing insulin-receptor expression (38). Vanadium is found in fish, vegetable oils, and olives. Excess vanadium supplementation should be avoided.

Diabetics often have low levels of magnesium, a mineral required for many physiological functions. People with the least amount of magnesium in their blood have twice the diabetes incidence as those with the highest levels. Scientists have shown that when magnesium-deficient patients were given supplements, their responsiveness to insulin and glucose metabolism improved (39). Fish, meat, seafood, and nuts are rich magnesium sources.

Other Supplements

The antioxidant alpha-lipoic acid is a common German treatment for diabetic neuropathy (antioxidants protect our bodies from cell-damaging, free radicals). Basically, with such neuropathy, persistent high blood-glucose generates oxidative stress that compromises blood flow to nerves, damaging signal-conducting axons. Over time, this damage may lead, for example, to foot problems requiring amputation. Through its antioxidant properties, alpha-lipoic acid enhances nerve health, lessening neuropathy (40). Red meat is a good source of alpha-lipoic acid.

The amino acid carnitine plays a key role in fat and glucose metabolism. Evidence suggests it lowers glucose levels through increasing glucose metabolism (i.e., burning it off) and creating glucose polymers called glycogen (i.e., putting it in storage). Double-blind clinical studies indicate that carnitine helps diabetic neuropathy by enhancing neuronal conduction and reducing pain (41). Beef is the richest source of carnitine.

The vitamin nicotinamide (a biochemical derivative of niacin) lowers blood-glucose levels by enhancing the pancreas' insulin-producing ability. For example, blood-glucose metabolism was improved in type-2 diabetics who had lost responsiveness to commonly prescribed sulfonylurea drugs (sulfonylureas make the pancreas release more insulin) after consuming nicotinamide for six months (42). Meat, fish, and poultry are good sources of this vitamin.

Foods and Botanical Medicines

Before insulin was developed, diabetes was treated throughout the world with a multitude of traditional plant remedies:

Ginseng is a traditional cure-all that restores a more health-promoting balance or homeostasis to the body. Studies show that diabetics who consumed American ginseng before an oral glucose challenge had lower blood-glucose levels (43). With such a challenge, fasting patients consume glucose, and then its elimination from the blood is followed over time. The results suggest that consuming ginseng before a meal could lower blood-sugar levels after the meal (i.e., postprandial).

Unripe *bitter melon*, a cucumber-shaped fruit, is a traditional Asian diabetes remedy (38). In one study, diabetics who drank juiced bitter-melon had lower fasting and postprandial blood-glucose levels. Bitter melon includes physiologically active agents that affect glucose metabolism, including an insulin-resembling molecule.

Gymnema, related to milkweed, is an Ayurvedic (India's ancient medicine) remedy for diabetes. Diabetics who consumed gymnema for 18 to 20 months had lower blood-sugar levels, and a significant number were able to discontinue conventional oral medications (44). In rats, gymnema doubled pancreatic, insulin-producing beta cells.

Fenugreek, a common Indian and Middle Eastern spice, possesses antidiabetic properties (45). In one study, diabetics who consumed fenugreek seed powder at lunch and dinner had substantially lower fasting-blood-glucose and demonstrated improved glucose-tolerance test results. Because fenugreek is somewhat bitter, it can also be taken in capsules available at health-food stores.

The pads and fruits of the *prickly pear cactus* or *nopal* are Hispanic foods that are also traditional antidiabetic remedies (46). Several studies demonstrate the ability of nopal, which contains substances that increase insulin sensitivity, to reduce blood-glucose levels in diabetics. Nopal can be consumed raw, cooked or juiced.

Another desert plant with antidiabetic properties is *aloe vera* (45). Best known as a topical remedy for burns and wounds, it is also a traditional Arabian Peninsula diabetes remedy. Studies suggest that diabetics who consume aloe gel daily over time can substantially lower blood-glucose levels.

Eating *nuts and nut butters* reduces diabetes risk, probably due to their fiber, healthy fats, and magnesium. In a nutshell, Harvard investigators followed 83,000 women and found that those who ate an ounce of nuts or a tablespoon of peanut butter five times a week or more reduced their risk of diabetes by nearly 30% (47).

Other potential antidiabetes foods include *noni juice* (Morinda citrifolia), a traditional Polynesian cure-all for many disorders; *cinnamon*; *jambul*, a plant related to cloves and another Ayurvedic remedy; and *stevia*, a popular sugar substitute isolated from a South American shrub.

Fiber

Evidence suggests that diabetes risk can be lowered by consuming dietary fibers that slow carbohydrate absorption, including *glucomannan*, a traditional Japanese food isolated from the konjac root (related to yams) (48); and *psyllium* (49), which is the laxative Metamucil's active ingredient.

Dietary Vices

Coffee addicts rejoice! Validating previous studies, Harvard investigators followed more than 126,000 subjects for up to 18 years and found that men who drank more than six cups (48 ounces) of coffee daily reduced their diabetes risk by more than 50% (30% for women) (50). The effect faded with fewer than three cups per day. Research suggests that coffee contains chemical that attenuate intestinal glucose absorption.

In addition, *moderate alcohol* consumption lowers diabetes risk, as it does for heart disease. For example, one study evaluated diabetes incidence in 23,000 Finnish twins (51). Results indicated that the twin who drank moderately but not heavily had half the diabetes risk as the twin who abstained or drank low amounts of alcohol. Among other mechanisms, moderate alcohol consumption may enhance insulin sensitivity. It goes without saying, however, that these diabetes-related benefits could be offset by other adverse effects.

Native-American Herbs

Native-American medicine emphasizes healing herbs, including many that target diabetes. According to *American Indian Healing Arts* (52), antidiabetic herbs include devil's club, barberry, uva ursi, Cananda and daisy fleabane, alum root, joe-pye weed, red trillium, wild ginger, clintonia, bugleweed, and flowering spurge. Extensive information on each of these herbs can be obtained through a Google Internet search (www.google.com).

Fats

Fat and carbohydrate metabolism are intimately connected, explaining why there are fat vegetarians and why people lose body fat on low-carbohydrate diets. As such, issues involving fat consumption and metabolism are of paramount importance in diabetes. One fat that is especially important is linolenic acid, an essential fatty acid that we must consume from our diet. Once consumed, we convert it to gamma-linolenic acid, an important precursor to prostaglandin hormones that regulate blood flow. This conversion is compromised in diabetics, which promotes diabetic neuropathy. Studies suggest that gamma-linolenic acid supplementation reduces such neuropathy (45). Primrose, borage, and black current oils are rich sources of this fatty acid.

One intriguing theory attributes diabetes development to the chronic consumption of bad fats and suggests that it can be cured by consuming good fats (53). This theory suggests that diabetes was relatively rare until the introduction of engineered fats into our food supply. Over time, these fats became a pervasive component of our diet and increasingly replaced the more natural fats that over eons our bodies had evolved physiologically to use. If sufficient amounts of unnatural fats intercalate into the cell membrane, membrane viscosity increases, compromising the ability of embedded insulin receptors to promote glucose uptake. It's like starting your car when it is 25 below and your engine still contains last summer's heavyweight oil. Turnover (i.e., glucose uptake) won't be that efficient. Conversely, if a diet is shifted to one that emphasizes more physiologically compatible fats, the bad fats would be eventually displaced from the membrane, once again enhancing receptor function.

Conclusions

With more than 200,000 Americans dying annually from a disease whose incidence continues to skyrocket, diabetes has become one of society's foremost health problems. Diabetes is the result of our long-term dietary and lifestyle choices; as a result, its management will depend on the shifts we make in these choices. Because individuals with SCI are predisposed to diabetes, they need to be especially disciplined in their choices. This chapter provides some nutritional and botanical options that may assist them in their efforts.

Additional Readings and Resources

Journals

Kliger B, Lynch D. An integrative approach to the management of type 2 diabetes mellitus. *Alternative Therapies* 2003; 9(6): 24–32.

Shane-McWhorter L. Biological complementary therapies: A focus on botanical products in diabetes. *Diabetes Spectrum* 2001; 14: 199–208.

Yarnell E. Southwestern and Asian botanical agents for diabetes mellitus. *Alternative and Complementary Therapies* 2000; 6(1): 7–11.

Yeh GY, Eisenberg DM, Kaptchuk TJ, et al. Systematic review of herbs and dietary supplements for glycemic control in diabetes. *Diabetes Care* 2003; 26: 1277–1294.

CREATING STRENGTH THROUGH CREATINE

If you wander through health-food stores, you may see muscular bodybuilders checking out creatine supplements. Many athletes now consume them to build strength and enhance athletic performance, especially for physical efforts requiring energy bursts. Ever since English Olympians initially brought attention to creatine's performance-enhancing benefits at the 1992 Barcelona games, creatine's popularity has skyrocketed. Its effectiveness is now supported by numerous scientific studies, including those suggesting benefits for people with physical disabilities, including spinal cord injury. Furthermore, animal studies indicate that creatine exerts a neuro-protective effect after injury.

Our bodies contain more than 100 grams of creatine (28 grams = 1 ounce), mostly in our muscles, heart, brain, and testes. Physical activity stimulates primarily the liver to produce about two grams of creatine daily from three key amino acids: glycine, arginine, and methionine. The creatine is then sent through the blood and transported into muscle cells. Creatine can also be provided by diet, especially one rich in meat and fish. Vegetarian diets, however, often lack not only creatine, but also the methionine precursor needed for internal production. For comparison's sake, a pound of meat contains about 40 times more creatine (two grams) than a pound of milk.

Creatine-Generated Energy

Most muscle creatine is converted into the energetically powerful creatine-phosphate. The high-energy molecular bond connecting the creatine to the phosphate group is an energy source that can quickly fuel muscle activity. This fueling, however, is mediated through the creation of yet another powerhouse molecule called adenosine triphosphate (ATP). ATP is extremely important because it is the body's energy currency, expended to drive most biochemical processes. Like creatine-phosphate, ATP's terminal phosphate group is connected by a high-energy bond that when severed provides energy needed for muscle contraction.

Under more constant or endurance working conditions, the body obtains ATP by metabolizing carbohydrates and fats, a relatively slow process that cannot generate immediately needed ATP energy. When energy bursts are required, the body uses creatine-phosphate instead. Specifically, the phosphate group on this molecule is transferred to replenish spent ATP, transforming it into its energetically powerful form. During rest periods, creatine-phosphate is then replenished by the ATP generated by the slower metabolic processes.

If intracellular creatine-phosphate levels can be increased, for example, through supplementation, it will take longer before the short-term energy source is depleted and a switchover to slower carbohydrate or fat metabolism is needed. This process can be visualized as if you have a large wad of cash (i.e., creatine-phosphate) in your wallet. It's there, ready to be used to meet your immediate needs. The more you supplement this wad, the more energy purchases you can make quickly. In contrast, generating your energy through carbohydrate or fat metabolism is the equivalent of writing a check that must clear the system, a more time-consuming process better suited to meet your long-term, larger needs.

Strength and Muscles

Creatine supplementation is most useful for physical activities that require intense bursts of energy, for example, a bench press, a sprint, or games requiring energy bursts. It is less useful for endurance events, except when such events are enhanced by building up muscle strength through creatine-stimulated weightlifting. Creatine can build muscle mass by several mechanisms. For example, because weightlifting is exactly the sort of short-term, intense physical activity fostered by creatine, more repetitions and harder workouts can be achieved, building up muscle. However, creatine also increases water uptake into the muscle, a process called cell volumizing that bulks up the muscles in a fashion that may not add much real strength.

Supplementation Cycle

In one commonly used, creatine-supplementation cycle, four 5-gram doses of creatine are consumed daily for five days. These are often dissolved in a sweetened solution to enhance uptake. After this loading phase, the daily dose is reduced to two grams for a month, after which supplementation is discontinued for an additional month. The cycle then starts over. The washout period is recommended because increased creatine levels will eventually trigger the body to shut down its creatine production and transport of the nutrient into muscle from the blood. After the washout period, the body regains these functions. Although some physical gains may be lost, the next cycle will start at a higher baseline because more intense workouts were achieved during the earlier supplementation phase.

Side Effects

In addition to potential transient gastrointestinal disturbances, chronic creatine supplementation may stress kidneys and increase exposure to potential manufacturing-process contaminants. Although risk appears low given its extensive history of use, normal metabolic patterns are affected to obtain the desired benefits, which over time may have yet undefined deleterious effects.

Physical Disability

Studies suggest that creatine can enhance strength compromised by physical disability. First, Dr. P. Jacobs and colleagues at the Miami Project have shown that creatine promotes upper-extremity work capacity in quadriplegics (54). In this study, 16 male quadriplegics with complete cervical C5-7 injuries were randomly assigned to receive either 20 grams/day of creatine or placebo maltodextrin (a common food ingredient) for seven days. Treatment was then discontinued for a three-week washout period, after which the treatment groups were reversed for another seven days; that is, the initial placebo group now received creatine, and the initial creatine group now was given maltodextrin. Work capacity was assessed before and after each dosing period using arm ergometry, a common SCI-rehabilitation exercise. Specifically, subjects faced a series of two-minute, increasing-intensity work stages with intervening one-minute recovery periods. After creatine supplementation, improvements were noted in various respiratory measurements, including oxygen uptake, carbon dioxide production, tidal volume (amount of air that enters the lungs), and breathing rate. For example, 14 of the 16 subjects demonstrated increased oxygen uptake, averaging a 19% improvement in uptake. Improvements were also noted in peak power output and increased time to fatigue.

Second, Dr. Kenneth Adams and colleagues of Dallas, Texas, carried out a creatine-loading study in 10 subjects with SCI (55). The subjects had their peak power production tested on an upper extremity exercise machine before and after creatine supplementation. Most improved their peak power production, with quadriplegics and paraplegics averaging 21% and 13% improvement respectively.

Third, doctors Stephen Burns and Rich Kendall (Seattle, Washington) have also evaluated the effects of creatine supplementation on arm strength in C-6 quadriplegics (personal communication, September 10, 2002). In this study, however, preliminary analyses indicated no major benefits. Burns speculates that creatine supplementation provides to both SCI and neurologically intact individuals similar modest benefits in response to repeated maximal efforts on short-duration exercises. However, these benefits may be offset by weight gains attributed to non-strength-associated water uptake. In other words, you may be hauling around more weight that will not enhance sporting or transfer ability.

Finally, doctors Mark Tarnopolsky and Joan Martin (Hamilton, Ontario) have shown that creatine can increase handgrip, knee-extension, and ankle strength in individuals with various forms of neuromuscular disease (56).

The differences in the indicated benefits among studies are not surprising because results can be affected by many interacting factors, including, in these cases, the selected outcome measures, dosing regimens, and sample sizes (e.g., more subjects may statistically demonstrate subtler effects).

Neuroprotective Effect

Animal studies indicate that creatine exerts a neuro-protective effect in traumatic brain and spinal cord injury. For example, Dr. O. Hausmann and colleagues of Zurich, Switzerland, demonstrated that four weeks of creatine supplementation before experimental spinal cord injury reduced glial scar formation and enhanced functional recovery in rats (57). In another example, Dr. A. Rabchevsky and colleagues (Lexington, Kentucky) showed that creatine supplementation spared spinal cord gray matter in injured rats (gray matter contains neuronal cell bodies and dendrites and glial cells; white matter consists mainly of axons) (58). These studies suggest that dietary supplementation with creatine may be a promising approach for reducing neurological damage after SCI.

Conclusions

Although more definitive studies are needed, creatine's potential benefits have important ramifications for many with SCI because the enhancement of residual strength, even to a limited degree, often can have profound quality-of-life implications. Furthermore, creatine supplementation may exert neuro-protective effects after acute spinal cord injury.

Additional Readings and Resources

Journals

Nick GL. Creatine phosphate complex and creatine serum. *Townsend Letter for Doctors and Patients* 2003; February/March: 160–165.

Books

Passwater RA. *Creatine.* New Canaan, Conn.: Keats Publishing, 1997.

Internet

Creatine Use during Exercise in Spinal Cord Injury (W. Young): http://carecure. rutgers.edu/spinewire/Articles/Creatine/creatine.htm

REFERENCES

1. *Prevention and Management of Urinary Tract Infections in Paralyzed Persons.* Agency for Health Care Policy and Research (AHCPR) Evidence Report/ Technology Assessment No 6 (AHCPR Publication No. 99-E008). Rockville, MD: U.S. DHHS.
2. Biering-Sorensen F, Bagi P, Hoiby N. Urinary tract infections in patients with spinal cord lesions: treatment and prevention. *Drugs* 2004; 61: 1275–1287.
3. Johnston LS, Neuhaus FC. Initial membrane reaction in the biosynthesis of peptidoglycan, spin-labeled intermediates as receptors for Vancomycin and Ristocetin. *Biochemistry* 1975; 14): 2754–2760.
4. Fisher JA. *The Plague Makers: How We Are Creating New Epidemics—And What We Must Do To Avert Them.* New York: Simon and Schuster, 1994.
5. Gilmore MS, Ferretti JJ. The thin line between gut commensal and pathogen. *Science* 2003; 299: 1999–2002.
6. Ferber D. WHO advises kicking the livestock antibiotic habit. *Science* 2003; 301: 1027.
7. Reid G, Hsiehl J, Potter P. Cranberry juice consumption may reduce biofilms on uroepithelial cells: pilot study in spinal cord injured patients. *Spinal Cord* 2001; 39: 26–30.
8. Schaeffer AJ, Chmiel JS, Duncan JL, et al. Mannose-sensitive adherence of Escherichia coli to epithelial cells from women with recurrent urinary tract infections. *J Urol* 1984; 131: 906–910.
9. Wright JV. D-mannose for bladder and kidney infections. *Townsend Letter for Doctors and Patients* 1999; 192: 96–98.

10. Wright JV, Lenard L. *D-Mannose and Bladder Infection: The Natural Alternative to Antibiotics.* Auburn, Wa.: Dragon Art, 2001.

11. D-mannose knocks pain and urgency from E. coli caused UTI's in 12-24 hours without antibiotics. *ACCM Health Sense* 2003; March: 1–4.

12. Balch PA. *Prescription for Herbal Healing.* New York: Penguin Putnam, 2002.

13. Keville K. *Aromatherapy for Dummies.* Foster City, Calif.: IDG Books Worldwide, 1999.

14. National Center for Homeopathy (www.homeopathic.org).

15. Grant WB. An ecologic study of dietary links to prostate cancer. *Altern Med Rev* 1999; 4(3): 162–169.

16. Gann PH, Ma J, Giovannucci E, et al. Lower prostate cancer risk in men with elevated plasma lycopene levels: results of a prospective analysis. *Cancer Res* 1999; 59: 1225–1230.

17. Giovannucci E, Rimm EB, Wolk A, et al. Calcium and fructose intake in relation of prostate cancer. *Cancer Res* 1998; 58: 442–447.

18. Clark LC, Dalkin B, Krongrad A, et al. Decreased incidence of prostate cancer with selenium supplementation: results of a double-blind cancer prevention trial. *Br J Urol* 1998; 81: 730–734.

19. Zhao X, Feldman D. The role of vitamin D in prostate cancer. *Steroids* 2001; 66:293–300.

20. Gunawardena K, Murray DK, Meikle AW. Vitamin E and other antioxidants inhibit human prostate cancer cells through apoptosis. *Prostate* 2000; 44: 287–295.

21. Sigounas G, Hooker J, Anagnostou A, et al. S-allymercaptocysteine inhibits cell proliferation and reduces the viability of erythroleukemia, breast, and prostate cancer cell lines. *Nutr Cancer* 1997; 27: 186–191.

22. Schoonen WM, Salinas CA, Kiemeney LA, et al, Alcohol consumption and risk of prostate cancer in middle-aged men. *Int J Cancer* 2004; 113: 133–140.

23. Murray MT. *The Healing Power of Herbs.* Rocklin, Calif.: Prima Publishing, 1995.

24. Breza J, Dzurny O, Borowka A, et al. Efficacy and acceptability of tadenan (Pygeum africanum extract) in the treatment of benign prostatic hyperplasia (BPH): a multicentre trial in central Europe. *Curr Med Res Opin* 1998; 14: 127–139.

25. Buck AC, Rees RWM, Ebeling L. Treatment of chronic prostatitis and prostatodynia with pollen extract. *Br J Urol* 1989; 64: 496–499.

26. Buck AC, Rees RWM, Ebeling L, et al. Treatment of outflow tract obstruction due to benign prostatic hyperplasia with the pollen extract, Cernilton: a double-blind, placebo-controlled study. *Br J Urol* 1990; 66: 398–404.

27. Dutkiewicz S., Usefulness of Cernilton in the treatment of benign prostatic hyperplasia. *Int Urol Nephrol* 1996; 28(1): 49–53.

28. Romics I. Observations with Bazoton in the management of prostatic hyperplasia. *Int Urol Nephrol* 1987; 19; 293–297.

29. Ullman D. *The Consumer's Guide to Homeopathy: The Definitive Resource for Understanding Homeopathic Medicine and Making it Work for You.* New York: Putnam, 1995.

30. Nachatelo M. Guilt-free sunbathing. *Natural Health* 2002; May/June: 54–57.

31. Luscombe CJ, Fryer AA, French ME, et al. Exposure to ultraviolet radiation: association with susceptibility age at presentation with prostate cancer. *Lancet* 2001; 358: 641–642.

32. John EM, Dreon DM, Koo J. Residential sunlight exposure is associated with a decreased risk of prostate cancer. *J Steroid Biochem Mol Biol* 2004; 89–90: 549–552.

33. Wennberg JE. Assessing therapies for benign prostatic hypertrophy and localized prostate cancer. *Agency for Health Care Policy and Research* (AHCPR) 1995; Available online at www.ahcpr.gov/clinic/medtep/bphport.htm

34. Bauman WA, Spungen AM. Disorders of carbohydrate and lipid metabolism in veterans with paraplegia or quadriplegia: A model of premature aging. *Metabolism* 1994; 43: 749–756.

35. Bauman WA, Adkins RH, Spungen AM, et al. The effect of residual neurological deficit on serum lipoprotein profiles in persons with chronic spinal cord injury. *Spinal Cord* 1998; 36: 13–17.

36. Bauman WA, Spungen AM, Wang J, et al. The relationship between energy expenditure and lean tissue in monozygotic twins discordant for spinal cord injury. *J Rehabil Res Dev* 2004; 41(1): 1–8.

37. Gilmore MS, Ferretti JJ. The thin line between gut commensal and pathogen. *Science* 2003; 299: 1999–2002.

38. Kliger B, Lynch D. An integrative approach to the management of type 2 diabetes mellitus. *Altern Ther Health Med* 2003; 9(6): 24–32.

39. Rodriguez-Moran M, Guerrero-Romero F. Oral magnesium supplementation improves insulin sensitivity and metabolic control in type 2 diabetic subjects: a randomized double-blind controlled trial. *Diabetes Care* 2003; 26: 1147–1152.

40. Ametov AS, Barinov A, Dyck PJ. The sensory symptoms of diabetic polyneuropathy are improved with alpha-lipoic acid: the SYDNEY trial. *Diabetes Care* 2003; 26:770–776.

41. De Grandis D, Minardi C. Acetyl-L-carnitine (levacecarnine) in the treatment of diabetic neuropathy. A long-term, randomized, double-blind, placebo-controlled study. *Drugs R D* 2002; 3: 223–231.

42. Polo V, Saibene A, Poniroli AE. Nicotinamide improves insulin secretion and metabolic control in lean type 2 diabetic patients with secondary failure to sulphonylureas. *Acta Diabetol* 1998; 35(1): 61–64.

43. Vuksan V, Starvo MP, Sievenpiper JL, et al. Similar postprandial glycemic reduction with escalation of dose and administration time of American ginseng in type 2 diabetes. *Diabetes Care* 2000; 23: 1221–1226.

44. Baskaran K, Kizar-Ahamath B, Radha-Shanmugasundaram K. Antidiabetic effect of a leaf extract from gymnema sylvestre in non-insulin-dependent diabetes mellitus patients. *J Ethanopharmaco* 1990; 30: 295–300.

45. Shane-McWhorter L. Biological complementary therapies: a focus on botanical products in diabetes. *Diabetes Spectrum* 2001; 14: 199–208.

46. Yarnell E. Southwestern and Asian botanical agents for diabetes mellitus. *Alternative and Complementary Therapies* 2000; 6(1): 7–11.

47. Jiang R, Manson JE, Stampfer MJ, et al. Nut and peanut butter consumption and risk of type 2 diabetes in women. *JAMA* 2002; 288: 2554–2560.

48. Chen HL, Sheu WH, Tai TS, et al. Konjac supplement alleviated hypercholesterolemia and hyperglycemia in type 2 diabetic subjects: a randomized double-blind trial. *J Am Coll Nutr* 2003; 22(1): 36–42.
49. Anderson JW, Allgood LD, Turner J, et al. Effects of psyllium on glucose and serum lipid responses in men with type 2 diabetes and hypercholesterolemia. *Am J Clin Nutr* 1999; 70: 466–473.
50. Salazar-Martinez E, Willett WC, Ascherio A, et al. Coffee consumption and risk for type 2 diabetes mellitus. *Ann Intern Med* 2004; 140(1): 1–8.
51. Carlsson S, Hammer N, Grill V, et al. Alcohol consumption and the incidence of type 2 diabetes: a 20-year follow-up of the Finnish twin cohort study. *Diabetes Care* 2003; 26: 2795–2790.
52. Kavash EB, Baar K. *American Indian Healing Arts: Herbs, Rituals, and Remedies for Every Season of Life.* New York: Bantam Books, 1999.
53. Smith T. Our deadly diabetes deception. *Nexus Magazine* 2004; July/August: 29–74. (Also www.healingmatters.com).
54. Jacobs PL, Mahoney ET, Cohn KA, et al. Oral creatine supplementation enhances upper extremity work capacity in persons with cervical-level spinal cord injury. *Arch Phys Med Rehabil* 2002; 83: 19–23.
55. Adams KK, Priebe M, Umoh D. The effects of creatine loading on the peak power production in patients with spinal cord injuries: A pilot study. *Arch Phys Med Rehabil* 2000; 81: 1263.
56. Tarnopolsky M, Martin J. Creatine monohydrate increases strength in patients with neuromuscular disease. *Neurology* 1999; 52: 854–857.
57. Hausmann ON, Fouad K, Wallimann T, et al. Protective effects of oral creatine supplementation on spinal cord injury in rats. *Spinal Cord* 2002; 40: 449–456.
58. Rabchevsky AG, Sullivan PG, Fugacci I, et al. Creatine diet supplement for spinal cord injury: Influences on functional recovery and tissue sparing in rats. *J Neurotrauma* 2003; 20: 659–669.

11

The Paradigm Expanding

INERT-GAS THERAPY: A NEW HEALING ENERGY FOR SPINAL CORD INJURY?

During my review of spinal cord injury (SCI) alternative medicine, I have come across many paradigm-expanding therapies that go much farther beyond mainstream biomedical thinking than those discussed in previous chapters. Although I could write an entire additional book on such therapies, I will conclude this book with a discussion of one of them.

Specifically, this chapter discusses inert-gas therapy and its supposed regeneration-catalyzing properties. In various permutations, inert-gas devices have been on the periphery of the alternative-medicine community for years but only recently seem to be gaining more visibility. They even have been incorporated into some physical-rehabilitation programs. Hockey players and others have used the devices in efforts to regenerate teeth. In a curious anecdotal case demonstrating their potential regenerative power (1), a man placed an inert-gas device next to his bed to promote healing of a deteriorated hip. His wife, who had undergone tubal cauterization to prevent further pregnancies, slept next to him. In an unintended side effect, the device apparently restored her reproductive capability over time, and she became pregnant.

Given the devices' regeneration-enhancing function, it has been suggested that they could provide the regenerative potential needed to mend an injured spinal cord.

Alternative Science

The scientific and mind–body–spirit theories behind these regeneration-enhancing devices are futuristic and thought-provoking in nature. Because the therapy is based on concepts far beyond the banks of the scientific mainstream (1), some preliminary discussion is required.

Inert-gas therapy's principles challenge our most sacrosanct beliefs on how the universe works, undercutting the foundation on which most scientists build. For example, the therapy is based upon the existence of a multidimensional, primary-energy source; the idea that we are fundamentally beings of energy, which determines our physical and biochemical makeup; and the assumption that our consciousness, including our thoughts, attitudes, emotions, and belief systems, interacts with our energetic nature to create our physical reality, including that associated with SCI. Although such propositions appear radical, they were in fact espoused throughout much of history and are being increasingly considered by some open-minded, prescient scientists.

Primary Energy

Inert-gas therapy is based on a concept that space is *something*, not *nothing* as most scientists believe. This something is called ether, which permeates all three of our dimensions and also higher dimensional space. Through interdimensional vortexes and gradients in this all-pervading ether, a primary energy ultimately becomes the source of all of our more familiar forces, such as electromagnetism, gravity, and nuclear forces, and, as indicated by Einstein's $E = mc^2$ equation, all mass that forms our physical reality. Because it is this primal energy in which the universe's antientropic, creative forces, including our individual and collective consciousness, are mediated through, it is not confined to scientific speculation, but has profound eschatological, cosmological, and spiritual significance.

Although etheric energy was a part of scientific thinking through much of history, in the 19th century, scientists started to develop alternative theories to explain how the universe works. These contemporary explanations have become ingrained in our scientific thinking, yet they don't always work unless the cards are stacked in their favor. Specifically, they can provide contradictory results, are unable to explain some of our most important physical phenomena, and cannot provide an all-encompassing, unifying theoretical framework. In contrast, etheric energy theory has the ability to explain it all and integrate the pieces. Although involving principles far beyond the scope of this book (1), it is postulated that higher-dimensional etheric energy is downloaded into more accessible and usable three-dimensional energy through *primary points.*

Inert Gas

One source of these powerful primary points is the nucleus of inert-gas elements, that is, helium, neon, argon, krypton, and xenon. Specifically, xenon is the most important one for creating the raw fuel energy for building regeneration potential in tissue, including potentially a traumatically injured spinal cord. When the energy generated by these primary points is accessed through the devices described below, the inert gases provide the raw fuel that our consciousness then can direct to create its physical manifestation.

In the periodic table, the inert gases are a unique elemental family. Helium is the lightest with a molecular weight of 4, and xenon is the heaviest with a molecular weight of 131. All are present in the air we breathe, ranging from the abundant argon and rare xenon at 7,600 and 0.036 parts per million, respectively. For illustration purposes, the average person will breathe in about 82 liters of argon and 0.39 milliliters (one thousandth of a liter) of xenon per day. Compared to other elements, the inert gases possess additional energy that keeps them in a higher vibrational, more gaseous state. Although elements of higher molecular weight tend to be liquids or solids, xenon and krypton—with molecular weights greater than iron, nickel, copper, and zinc—exist as gases. This requires them to be in a higher vibrational state, which requires additional energy.

Helium also has properties that run counter to what would be expected when compared to other elements. Specifically, helium is difficult to freeze no matter how low the temperature is taken. Even if virtually all the thermal energy is removed, helium somehow retains sufficient vibrational energy that inhibits it from entering a solid state. Several years ago, I met the physicist who received the Nobel Prize for demonstrating this phenomenon.

It is postulated that primary points located in the nucleus of the inert-gas elements produce the energy that keeps the heavier inert-gas elements in a gaseous state and keeps helium from solidifying at very low temperatures. To harness the energy produced by these inert-gas primary points, devices have been constructed in which the inert-gas mixtures are electromagnetically stimulated. This stimulation pulls the primary point away from its nucleus, which under normal conditions would absorb the downloaded, primary-point energy. Because of this unshielding, the energy is now released into the surrounding space, and hence is available for healing purposes.

In one device, a sufficiently strong magnetic field is applied to a nonmagnetic metal chamber containing a pressurized inert-gas mixture (e.g., 25 times atmospheric pressure). In another less powerful, but more convenient and inexpensive device, the inert-gas mixture and a small magnet are enclosed within an airtight, Pyrex-glass capsule (about $1^1/_2$ by $^1/_4$ inch) under relatively low pressure. These inert-gas pendants can be readily placed at the point of injury, for example, worn around the neck or held close to some other body area.

Human Energy Fields

To understand inert-gas healing, we must review concepts of human-energy fields. Under such concepts, we are primarily beings of energy, which determines our physical, biochemical, and physiological nature. Energy fields (also called energy or subtle body, among others terms) that surround and permeate our physical body define much our energetic nature. When these energy fields are factored in, our physical body represents only a small component of who we are. As discussed by neurophysiologist Dr. Valerie Hunt, sophisticated, state-of-the-art technology can detect these fields (2). Interestingly, what is detected correlates well to what is observed independently by sensitive intuitives. This technology, however, only detects the lower-vibrational electromagnetic components of our fields, which range from these components to the powerful etheric forces discussed previously.

In *Hands of Light*, Barbara Brennan explains how the human energy field is composed of at least seven consecutive layers of increasing vibrational energy (3). Intersecting the body and the energy field are seven tornado-like energy vortexes, in Eastern traditions called chakras, which convert high vibrational energy into energy the body can assimilate. Our energy network includes a power column, in front of the spinal cord, which receives energy from the chakras and transmits it vertically through the body. A spinal cord injury decreases the energy flow through the body because of the cord's proximity to the power column and because the energy received by the lower chakras is reduced. The more familiar acupuncture points and meridians are further down our energetic pipeline, bringing downloaded energy to a more specific organ level.

Basically, the physical body is the lowest vibrational state of our energetic self. As a rough comparison, envision our energy fields as a set of Russian nesting dolls in which the smallest doll is enclosed by a larger one, and that doll by one larger still. The smallest innermost doll represents our physical body.

Imbalances or blockages in your energy network will predispose you to illness. Basically, disease has its origins in the energy field, which then progressively manifests at the molecular, cellular, and body-system levels. The energy field responds to stimulus even though you experience no conscious awareness of the stimulus and before changes are noted in physiological parameters such as brain waves, blood pressure, and so forth. Based on this presaging, technology can measure and assess energy disturbances in the field long before the onset of physical disease.

The Body Double

Under human-energy-field theories, every part of the physical body has a higher vibrational component (called para) within the energy field, such as the para-brain, para-eyes, para-bones, para-skin, and para-spinal cord. Specifically, the field closest to the body contains the body's template, duplicating every cell and organ. Because the physical body interacts with its higher vibrational version, as an acute spinal-cord injury evolves over time into a chronic injury, the distorted physical will be imprinted onto the higher-level-energy template. This locks the injury more into place, and as a result it becomes much more difficult for healing to take place by exclusively focusing on the physical. This represents a fundamental limitation in our conventional Western medicine. It is like trying to push a car in one direction when the steering wheel is cranked for another direction. In contrast, energy workers attempt to minimize these energetic barriers to physiological healing in SCI by mending the field's dysfunctional energy vectors.

Consciousness and Energy Fields

In addition to duplicating our physical bodies, the higher-vibrational energy fields are the repository for our consciousness. Our brain is a mere physiological processor for this consciousness. Although possessing a good processor affects your overt intelligence, and although outward expression of consciousness may be a function of your brain's neurons, complexity of synaptic connections, and so forth, it is not the site of your consciousness anymore than your big toe is. Again, under human-energy-field theories, all attributes of consciousness, such as your thoughts, attitudes, emotions, and perceptions, are stored in your energy fields. It is important to understand this conceptually, because your belief systems determine whether you can productively access and direct the inherently neutral, inert-gas primary energy for healing purposes, including spinal cord regeneration.

Pulling the Pieces Together

Our para-DNA, the higher-vibrational reflection of our genetic DNA, possesses the informational patterns to create a complete and whole physical body, including regenerating damaged components such as an injured spinal cord. Basically, this regenerative potential can be manifested in the physical if (a) sufficient etheric energy, the raw fuel of creation, can be built up in our energy fields and (b) pervasive negative belief systems (e.g., "you will never walk again") that prevent para-DNA-encoded vibrational information from being transferred into the physical are dismantled and replaced with beliefs of healing and renewed wholeness.

Inert-gas devices, especially those containing xenon, can help build up the etheric raw fuel needed for regeneration. In itself, however, this etheric fuel is neutral. Like the amorphous clay that is transformed into a work of art through the potter's consciousness, it is the directed consciousness of wholeness that will create its physical manifestation. Negative belief patterns that are hard to let go and that hang around in the energy fields will strongly filter these potent healing energies from reaching the physical. Essentially, the supplemental etheric energy facilitates the transference of the appropriate patterns held within the para-DNA into the physical structures. The intervening material is the energy body. The inert-gas devices are producing the specific raw material that the physical body will draw upon that is most advantageous to the healing process.

The energy fields are using the etheric energy as a means of communication that goes back and forth from nonphysical vibrational levels into the physical and back to the nonphysical. If a sufficient excess of etheric energy is available and can be appropriately directed, there is a spillover that will generally move into the body's weakest areas.

Meditative Visualization

To direct the nonspecific inert-gas energy to where it is needed, meditative visualization is required, for example, focusing on where the spinal dislocation has occurred, the nerves that need to be mended, and the bone that needs to be changed. A focus on the physical anatomy will be more helpful for those with a logical mind orientation. Those with a more intuitive mind orientation should perceive this anatomy symbolically as a landscape to be healed, as energy to be channeled into a large sculpture of the body. For most individuals, the translation from the etheric to physical level will take at least six months. In other words, if you meditate on seeing the body whole and healed, the additional etheric energy may be more readily transmitted about six months down the road into something physical.

An Inert-Gas Protocol for SCI

The following represents one specific inert-gas therapeutic protocol that has been provided to me for SCI. In this protocol, it is recommended that therapy begin with a pendant device containing an inert-gas combination emphasizing xenon (e.g., 46% xenon, 18% helium, 36% neon; see sources listed below). This combination can build energy in the spine. In the time of the waxing moon, alternate this combination with pure xenon or pure helium. If you are young (that is, with lots of regenerative forces), use pure helium. The reason for doing it during the waxing phase of the moon is that astronomical and geophysical influences on our biology are well documented. Although often overwhelmed by our pervasive electromagnetic environment (for example, computer monitors, cell phones, etc.), our physiology is very sensitive to the rhythmic or cyclic energy dynamics of the universe we live in, including lunar cycles. Virtually all therapeutic interventions, including pharmaceuticals and surgeries, are affected by such geophysical cycles.

In addition to the visualizations mention above, let sleep be deep. Let there be an attunement to dreams, lucid dreaming, and whatever your belief patterns can orient towards for bringing up issues and the understanding of new awareness.

During the waning moon, alternate the initial mixture with an argon and krypton combination (e.g., 96% argon and 4% krypton). This combination is especially useful to blow apart belief patterns; to dismantle old thought forms; and to examine why there might be issues of hopelessness, shame, or other negative emotions associated with the healing process. Byron Katie's methods are especially useful for the dismantling of old belief patterns (4).

Inert-gas energies can be transmitted in a variety of other ways. For example, they are carried well by water and can be taken in by drinking or bathing in water that has been exposed to the devices. Also, it is possible for energy workers or healers to absorb the energy, allowing it to move through their bodies and then their clients'.

Overdosing with inert-gas energy is possible; symptoms include sleeplessness, nervousness, and agitation. However, by stopping the application, you can rapidly recover and begin using it again at a lower level. I was affected personally by such inert-gas overdosing. While helping a colleague ascertain the influence of a relatively powerful inert-gas device (not the small pendants) on my energy fields as measured by another sophisticated machine, I repeatedly exposed myself to inert-gas energy. Although normally I can barely stay awake past 10 p.m., that night I stayed up much of the night, writing an article with rapidity and lucidity, which is usually a slow process for me.

Inert-gas therapy will have the greatest impact on individuals who are in the most nutritionally strong state. In addition to introducing etheric energy and busting apart the energy-filtering belief patterns, you need the nutritional building blocks necessary to regenerate a spinal cord. Specifically, consuming the right sort of fats will be an especially important for regenerating lipid-rich neuronal tissue (5).

Conclusions

Inert-gas technology is a new concept for building up regenerative energy after spinal cord injury. Although its potential theoretically would be relatively easy to test scientifically using active and placebo devices, the technology defies the scientific status quo. However, if you study the lessons of history, there is one scientific truth: today's cutting-edge insights are inevitably tomorrow's anachronisms. Reflecting this truth, it is worth repeating the words of one of history's most prominent physicians, Paracelsus (1493–1541), who stated, "That which is looked upon by one generation as the apex of human knowledge is often considered an absurdity by the next, and that which is regarded as a superstition in one century, may form the basis of science for the following one."

With relatively innocuous inert-gas therapy, you have nothing to lose, except perhaps the self-defeating beliefs that are obscuring the vision of your wholeness gathering on the horizon.

Sources

Inert-gas pendants can be obtained from Pegasus Products, Boulder, CO (www.pegasusproducts.com). The VIBE machine (www.vibe machine.com) is another, very different inert-gas device I have observed (it is similar to the one that kept me up all night).

Additional Readings and Resources

Books

Brennan BA. *Hands of Light: A Guide to Healing Through the Human Energy Field.* New York: Bantam Books, 1988.

Cooke MB. *Einstein Doesn't Work Here Anymore: A Treatise on the New Science.* Toronto: Marcus Books, 1983.

Hunt VV. *Infinite Mind: Science of the Human Vibrations of Consciousness.* Malibu, Calif.: Malibu Publishing, 1996.

REFERENCES

1. Cooke MB. *Einstein Doesn't Work Here Anymore: A Treatise on the New Science.* Toronto: Marcus Books, 1983.

2. Hunt VV. *Infinite Mind: Science of the Human Vibrations of Consciousness.* Malibu, Calif.: Malibu Publishing, 1996.

3. Brennan BA. *Hands of Light: A Guide to Healing Through the Human Energy Field*. New York: Bantam Books, 1988.
4. The Work of Byron Katie (www.thework.com).
5. Vonderplanitz A. *We Want To Live*. Santa Monica, Calif.: Carnelian Bay Castle Press, 1997.

Index